Manifesting Happy

Manifesting Happy

How to Maintain Self-Care Amid Challenging Behaviors and Challenging Times

Jenna Sage

ROWMAN & LITTLEFIELD
Lanham • Boulder • New York • London

Published by Rowman & Littlefield
An imprint of The Rowman & Littlefield Publishing Group, Inc.
4501 Forbes Boulevard, Suite 200, Lanham, Maryland 20706
www.rowman.com

Copyright © 2021 by Jenna Sage

All rights reserved. No part of this book may be reproduced in any form or by any electronic or mechanical means, including information storage and retrieval systems, without written permission from the publisher, except by a reviewer who may quote passages in a review.

British Library Cataloguing in Publication Information Available

Library of Congress Cataloging-in-Publication Data

Names: Sage, Jenna, 1977- author.
Title: Manifesting happy : how to maintain self-care amid challenging behaviors and challenging times / Jenna Sage.
Description: Lanham : Rowman & Littlefield, [2021] | Includes bibliographical references. | Summary: "The book contains self-care strategies to practice and even ideas to implement with students"—Provided by publisher.
Identifiers: LCCN 2020057565 (print) | LCCN 2020057566 (ebook) | ISBN 9781475856743 (cloth) | ISBN 9781475856750 (pbk) | ISBN 9781475856767 (ele)
Subjects: LCSH: Teachers—Mental health. | Teaching—Psychological aspects. | Stress management. | Well-being. | Self-care, Health.
Classification: LCC LB2840 .S34 2021 (print) | LCC LB2840 (ebook) | DDC 371.102—dc23
LC record available at https://lccn.loc.gov/2020057565
LC ebook record available at https://lccn.loc.gov/2020057566

This book is dedicated to every single hardworking, compassionate, essential educator. You are champions and heroes.

If the environment stays the way it is now then the bodily conditions will stay as they are and the feelings of those conditions will remain unchanged.

—B. F. Skinner Grandfather of
Applied Behavior Analysis

Contents

Acknowledgments	xiii
Introduction	1
1 *Metanoia*—Greek: *Self-Care and the Journey to Changing One's Mind*	3
What Is Self-Care?	3
Why Is Self-Care Important for Educators?	4
Eight Dimensions of Self-Care	5
Balancing Act	12
Self-Care Synergy	14
Notes	14
2 *Prajna*—Sanskrit: *Insights into Applied Behavior Analysis*	17
What Is Applied Behavior Analysis?	17
Classical Conditioning	17
Operant Conditioning	19
Forming Habits	20
ABCs of Behavior	21
Reinforcement and Punishment	24
Schedules of Reinforcement	27
Self-Care Synergy	28
Notes	29

3	*Acora Imparo*—Italian: *Wellness in the Learning Space*	31
	Habits in the Classroom	31
	Applied behavior analysis in the Classroom	32
	Classroom Connections	33
	Self-Care Synergy	35
4	*Ikigai*—Japanese: *Understanding the Reason for Being*	37
	Understanding Why	37
	Functions of Behavior	38
	Working Together	41
	Self-Care Synergy	42
5	*Amat Victoria Curam*—Latin: *Planning and Preparation for Self-Care*	45
	Planning for Self-Care	45
	Discover	46
	Self-Care Synergy	48
6	*Kujichagulia*—African: *Creating and Defining Self-Care*	49
	Define	49
	Self-Care Synergy	60
7	*Eunoia*—Greek: *Designing a Well-Balanced Self-Care Plan*	61
	Design	61
	Sensory Activities	62
	Escape/Avoid Activities	65
	Attention Activities	67
	Tangible Activities	69
	Self-Care Synergy	72
	Note	73
8	*Meraki*—Greek	75
	Do	75
	Self-Care Synergy	78
	Note	78
9	*Kalo*—Hawaiian: *Self-Care for Students*	79
	Paying It Forward	79
	Candle Blowout	79

Crossing the Meridian	80
Proprioceptive Positions	80
Tuck like an Armadillo	81
Countdown to Calm	81
Self-Care Synergy	82
Notes	83
Conclusion	**85**
Self-Care Is a Practice	85
Be Observant	86
Be Flexible	87
Be Diligent	87
Be Patient	88
Be Kind	88
Appendix	**89**
Endnote References	**97**
About the Author	**99**

Acknowledgments

I would like to acknowledge my mom, the first educator that truly touched my life, who retired from teaching after more than thirty years of service and thousands of lives touched. Thank you for being an inspiration.

I would like to acknowledge Stephanie Martinez, who is not only one of the kindest humans but also one of the best educators I know. Thank you for helping to review and edit this book with me.

I must thank my amazing husband, who knows every fit and start on my writing journey. Thank you for knowing me so well, for pushing me so much, for wiping away tears and for laughing alongside me. I could never be who I am without you.

Thanks to my dad and my brother, who have been amazing teachers to me in the classroom that we call life.

Most importantly, thanks to every single person who has dedicated their life to the service of others, whether you are a teacher, administrator, support personnel, caregiver, healthcare professional, or a volunteer. Thank you.

Introduction

In late February and early March of 2020, the need for and the conversation surrounding "self-care" for educators shifted. We found ourselves in the midst of a viral pandemic. Suddenly the world was forced to migrate inside. We had to quarantine and practice a new way of life that was at a distance from others. This found us mandated. We had to stay at home.

The field of education was forced to make a rapid and progressive change to the delivery of instruction from afar. Schools were closed. Classrooms empty. Children stayed at home, and, in most cases, parents had to assist with delivering remote learning.

Teachers literally had to modify their lessons, content, and activities to online platforms or distance learning. Parents had to adjust to being a facilitator of learning. And everyone had to create a new sense of normal.

It is most often in times of uncertainty, in times of duress that people learn their capacity to adapt and become agile. As Charles Darwin stated, "It is not the strongest of the species that survive, nor the most intelligent, but the one most responsive to change." So, collectively, the world changed.

The narrative about self-care changed too. The morning news, every social media platform, neighbors, and grandparents began talking about the need for self-care. More than ever, and in some instances, for the first time, people valued mental health and wellness.

Understandably too. For the first time in our lifetime, millions of people were forced to isolate themselves. People were unable to visit family, socialize at local restaurants, or interact with coworkers. There is a toll that isolation takes on our mental health, and there is a price paid for coping with the crisis.

As I continued to write this book, it began to feel disingenuous. How could I write a book about everyday life in the classroom when, if even temporary, everyday life in the classroom no longer existed? How could I be the expert on self-care among the hundreds of others out there sharing tips and strategies?

And then I remembered: educators are *always* educators. Whether they are in their classroom, in the hallways of a school, or sitting in their living room, teachers are steadfast in being committed to their students and to their mission of learning. I had to be steadfast too.

This book is going to offer something different than just tips on how to exercise more or eat healthy foods. It is going to go beyond sharing yoga positions or guided meditations. Though each of those strategies could be the right fit for you, this book is going to help you identify the best way to care for yourself and to nurture your mental health and well-being.

While this viral crisis may be temporary, the challenges of the classroom are constant. The stressors and the pressures are still there. The need for educators to care for themselves will always be needed.

Before this pandemic, educators faced the scrutiny of standardized assessments. Educators experienced criticism from families and the media. Teachers faced long hours, low wages, and under-appreciation.

While some of that has shifted due to the COVID-19 pandemic of 2020, educators will always have one of the most difficult jobs out there. Educators will continue to pour themselves into their work. They will continue to absorb the difficulties their students experience. Teachers will suffer from vicarious trauma. They will nurture the most challenging student.

If there is one thing that a worldwide focus on education has done, it is providing more appreciation for the field of education and for the science of teaching. As parents around the globe worked to organize, plan, and provide instruction, the understanding of the struggles that teachers face became more apparent. Parents and politicians finally had better insight into just how demanding teaching can be.

Together now, we can all move forward toward a new "way of work." Together as families, communities, and colleagues, we can support each other in being our happiest selves. Now, more than ever, we need to manifest happy.

Chapter 1

Metanoia—Greek

The journey of changing one's mind, heart, or way of life; spiritual conversion.

Self-Care and the Journey to Changing One's Mind

WHAT IS SELF-CARE?

There are numerous definitions of self-care. Ultimately, self-care is one of the activities that you engage in to maintain a healthy mental and physical presence. Searching online for self-care strategies or chatting with friends about what they do to care for themselves can result in mixed messages or multiple suggestions. If you are a person starting a self-care journey, that can feel overwhelming.

The search for a self-care routine shouldn't feel forced or overwhelming, but it will indeed be a journey. Self-care often requires establishing new habits and routines. This book is intended to help on the self-care journey by using a scientific approach.

By applying the science of behavior to self-care you will be able to better identify what strategies will work best for you. Out of the millions of ideas floating around on the Internet, this book will help to narrow down the search to those strategies that fit your needs best.

Applied behavior analysis is a science often applied in school settings and utilized by educators. Later, you'll learn more about practical applications and revisit lessons from the psychology 101 courses and human development courses you likely took. For now, let's understand self-care in more detail.

Self-care has been analogized as "putting your oxygen mask on first," "you can not pour from an empty cup," "you wouldn't let your phone battery go uncharged, why do it to yourself?" All of those analogies have one thing in common. You! You are the key to self-care. Self-care is about putting your needs in front of the needs of others.

That is not something easily done, especially for educators. As teachers, or administrators, or support personnel, we are drawn to the field of education to be a helper, a nurturer, and a guide. Educators are some of the most selfless people out there. Self-care can feel selfish, especially to educators, and they may feel compelled to shy away from it when, in reality, focusing on themselves is the first step to caring for those they intend to help.

WHY IS SELF-CARE IMPORTANT FOR EDUCATORS?

The concept of teacher burnout is nothing new. For the past two decades, there has been an increased focus within education about the rate at which teachers leave the profession. In Japanese culture burnout is called *karoshi* or "overwork death." It is a way to explain the way we over-dedicate ourselves to work to the degree that it negatively impacts our health and wellness.

- Nearly 44 percent of beginning teachers leave the profession within the first five years.[1]
- Fifty percent of teachers reported considering quitting or leaving the profession.[2]
- Nineteen percent directly linked the desire to quit with stress, burnout, and pressure.[3]

For educators that work with specific vulnerable populations (e.g., students with disabilities) those numbers can increase. The stress of working with difficult students, a lack of community support, increased pressures for performance outcomes on standardized assessments, a lack of academic freedom, being exposed to vicarious trauma and facing long hours, financial burdens due to underpaying, and being under-resourced can understandably take its toll.

Many educators enter the field, knowing it is a challenging profession. They experience the "call to teach." They have a desire to help, they have a passion for sharing knowledge, they have subject matter expertise, they have a deep well of compassion to share, and they love watching their students grow and learn. Whether novice teachers entering the field, experienced educators transitioning through more administrative roles, or career changers looking for a new passion, educators are traditionally selfless by nature.

Self-care becomes increasingly important for educators so they can sustain and maintain that passion and compassion. The statistics of burnout and educators leaving the profession occur primarily because of the inability to sustain the passion for long periods of time due to a lack of support. Think of it as a mathematical equation. For every year of passion poured into the profession it may take twice that in strategic self-care input to maintain.

Think about the analogy from earlier. You can't pour from an empty cup. When your morning coffee begins to empty, you pour more coffee into it. But for ourselves, we often neglect to continue to give back as much as we give out. For many, it is not for lack of wanting to care for ourselves, but it is a lack of time, energy, and/or knowledge. At the end of long days, it is hard to dedicate anything back to oneself.

EIGHT DIMENSIONS OF SELF-CARE

To better prepare for finding the best self-care strategy to meet your needs, let's review the different dimensions of self-care. Health and wellness have long been in the realm of physicians. The focus of patient wellness was predominately on healing the body, reacting to symptoms, and attempting to ameliorate them.

Around the 1970s, after years of people being deemed mentally ill and being prescribed heavy medication dosages, a movement occurred: a focus on the mind-body connection. A deliberate movement to move away from Western medicine and adopt more Eastern medical and prevention frameworks for health resulted in a holistic approach, and alternative focus was born.

The 1980s brought us home exercise plans and a fitness focus. The 1990s began a health movement for those that could afford wheatgrass and sustainable farm-to-table foods. Eventually, in the 2000s, health and wellness became household activities. More people not only had access to yoga classes and mobile applications to help take deep breaths, but self-care became mainstream. More people planned days to spend at the masseuse or spa. The use of

Table 1.1 Eight Dimensions of Wellness

Intellectual
Physical
Environmental
Financial
Occupational
Spiritual
Social
Emotional

chiropractic care and healthy vitamins and supplements increased. A health and wellness revolution was heightened, and self-care was the main theme.

One component of understanding and beginning the self-care journey is working toward balance (table 1.1). The Substance Abuse and Mental Health Services Administration (SAMHSA)[4] has defined eight dimensions of wellness. While each dimension serves to help build an overall sense of health and wellness, each individual should set a goal to find balance. In future chapters, as you build your comprehensive self-care plan, you'll want to deepen the depth of your wellness balance.

In order to create balance, first you must learn about all the dimensions that impact your well-being. Those dimensions are intellectual, physical, environmental, financial, occupational, spiritual, social, and emotional. This will be a brief introduction to the dimensions as future chapters continue to build out additional layers of learning.

Intellectual

Intellectual well-being is about staying informed. Many educators especially consider themselves to be lifelong learners and to engage in intellectual exercises. This dimension is about keeping your brain engaged and active.

Just like physical exercise you can plateau if you don't change up your routine. For anyone that has tried to lose weight or train for a physical event, you know that you can't engage in the same physical activity and get the best results. You have to target specific muscle groups and engage different parts of the body.

The brain is a muscle. The same way that your muscles can either atrophy with no use or stagnate with the same routine, your brain will do the same thing. The brain requires assistance to develop new neural pathways to grow stronger.

Practice this activity:

1. Stand up.
2. Shake your arms.
3. Cross your arms in your most comfortable and confident "arms crossed teacher pose"—feels good, right?
4. Now, uncross your arms and shake them out again.
5. Cross your arms in the opposite direction/pattern—it feels different, doesn't it?

Take a moment to reflect. Why did the first time feel comfortable? Was it more difficult the second time, in a pattern that wasn't as familiar? Why do you think that is?

Your arms create muscle memory. Most people have a dominant side of their body, and from an early age, they favor that side when crossing their arms or legs to the point that doing it in a different way can make us feel uncomfortable.

The same way that your muscles create memory, the pathways, the neural connections in your brain also develop "comfortable patterns." Most people don't stretch their brain beyond what is necessary, while other people love stretching their brain-power.

As educators there are opportunities for professional development, staying active with associations and organizations, and extended personal learning opportunities through critical thinking and problem-solving activities. The goal won't have to be learning a new language or a new skill, though it certainly could; it will simply require finding ways to keep your mind active and engaged in ways that help to stretch your brain-power.

Physical

Similarly, your body needs to gain strength and power as well. You don't have to become a body-builder and don't even necessarily have to set a goal to lose weight, but you do want to focus on your physical well-being, on feeling good, and on having a positive body relationship.

Physical well-being includes sleep patterns, eating patterns, and understanding how movement and stillness can impact you. As teachers, you are likely on your feet for most of the day. You likely have few opportunities to rest your body during the day. How then do you find balance at times to be still?

Physical well-being is also about your medical wellness. Whether you are in perfect health or have chronic or ongoing medical concerns, your physical health is impacted by the care you place on your medical health. Do you regularly take necessary medications? Do you engage in alternative medical practices? Do you generally feel healthy? Do you want to feel less pain or more muscle movement?

Developing your balanced self-care plan will require that you consider goals for your physical health as much as your mental health. With the mind-body connection, it is difficult to impact one without the other. Much the way, it is difficult to impact only behavior or only academics in the classroom. The two go hand in hand.

Environmental

Do you enjoy the sound of the rain on the rooftop or the smell of salty air rolling off the beach? Environmental wellness is both enjoying the natural

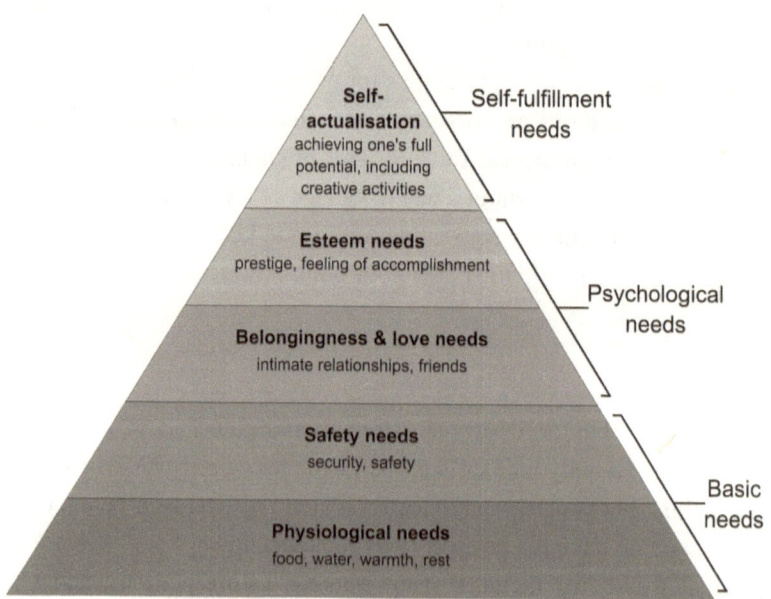

Figure 1.1 **Maslow's Hierarchy of Needs.** *Original Source*: https://en.wikipedia.org/wiki/Maslow%27s_hierarchy_of_needs

surroundings and having safe access to what nature can provide. Clean water, safe home and work environments, and sustainable resources help create well-being.

In education there is a popular saying, "Maslow[5] before Bloom." This suggests that basic needs have to be met before psychological needs (figure 1.1).

Those basic physiological and safety needs are key foundational pieces to building a wellness and self-care plan. Have you ever had a student in your classroom that was incredibly difficult to teach, a student who was hypersensitive or hyper-aroused? Perhaps a student who was unkempt or had poor hygiene habits? Students whose basic needs have not been met, who live in unstable conditions or go without food can oftentimes appear to lack motivation or be unwilling or even unable to learn. But it may just be that their basic safety and physiological needs have not been met, so they are not cognitively ready for learning.

Being able to access safety and security is part of the environmental dimension, so is being one with nature, enjoying nature. For the nature lovers and gardeners out there, research has even shown that there are microbes in the soil that can act as antidepressants.[6] You may not be the hands-in-the-dirt kind of person and that is fine. But you may want to consider additional opportunities to engage with nature and experience the natural world. That may look like observing the wind in the trees or watching clouds make new shapes. It may look like walks through parks, preserves, or neighborhood co-op gardens. To appreciate nature, you don't have to become a naturalist, but you can find opportunities to become closer to nature in safe and secure ways.

Financial

Another fundamental wellness area is financial. In families, many arguments, stressors, and complications arise over finances. Having a steady income, savings for emergencies, and the ability to plan for and enjoy retirement or extra activities can impact feelings of financial security.

You can even go so far as to think of your own self-care and wellness as a bank account that you want to grow. Just like you learn saving and spending behaviors, you also learn self-care and wellness behaviors. You want to take this opportunity to begin to adjust your habits and routines to save for your financial account and your wellness account.

The adage that money doesn't bring happiness is often true. The statement by the rapper Notorious B.I.G. "mo money, mo problems" is also often true. Financial wellness is about finding the level of security that makes sense for you and your family. You may not need excess and you may be satisfied with having little. You may be a saver or you may be a spender. For financial wellness, like all of the dimensions, it is about balance.

Occupational

Similarly, occupational wellness springs from a sense of security with one's job. It also involves enjoyment, passion, and purpose with your job. As educators, many of you likely entered the field with a sense of purpose to help, a desire to improve lives and make a difference. In any job, that passion can begin to wilt or shift. Finding occupational wellness is important to sustain that passion and work against the stressors that can create burnout and dissatisfaction.

Occupational wellness can also include the balance between your career and other activities to ensure that time is devoted to the other dimensions of wellness in a strategic way. It can also represent opportunities to find personal satisfaction and motivation within your job. Education can often feel like a thankless profession, so it is vital as part of occupational wellness to focus on areas of appreciation within your job.

Spiritual

Spirituality is often connected to faith and a belief in a higher power or being. In this wellness dimension though, it is about general beliefs and value systems. This dimension of wellness is about providing yourself time to engage in purpose-finding and making sense of your greater purpose.

You can choose to incorporate religion, faith, and spiritual beliefs, or you might choose to focus on appreciation for life and how you fit into the natural world. Spirituality, in this case, is about making meaning as a human within context of the greater universe and surroundings.

For many, spirituality is about hope or trust in a universal path, a divine guidance. For others, spirituality may look agnostic or skeptical. It may be an appreciation of the sciences. And for some, spirituality may even include conspiracies and other-worldly beliefs. For spiritual wellness, it is important to engage in practices that support a value system that promotes personal health and, if possible, peace and harmony.

Social

The social dimension is likely one you feel most familiar with. As an educator, you likely spend a great deal of time focused on healthy socialization in your school and classroom. You likely also work on having healthy personal relationships and establishing opportunities for engaging in social activities inside and outside of the school setting.

Humans are naturally social creatures. Most people, if forced to isolate themselves from others, will experience a sense of loss, grief, stress, and diminished mental wellness. Some people may not always feel comfortable in large groups of people, but having a connection to other people is important.

You might recall the theories of Albert Bandura, which surmise that humans learn from each other through observation and modeling. As you learn more about applied behavior analysis in the next chapter, you will see psychology theorists continued to build on that model to better understand human behavior.

What we do know is that from our earliest interactions with another human, we are learning and most often we are learning because of a reciprocal interaction between two or more people. Learning most often requires other humans. As an educator, you play a fundamental role in that learning and providing opportunities to create healthy social opportunities.

Social emotional learning (SEL) has gained significant popularity in classrooms across the nation. The increasing educational focus on Maslow's hierarchy and the acknowledgment that there is an inseparable connection between academics and behaviors, much the way it is difficult to separate mind from body, has allowed for educators to address the social and emotional needs of students along with the academic needs.

Emotional

The emotional dimension was intentionally left for last. This dimension tends to be the one that lets you know if any other dimension is significantly out of balance. When emotions become out of balance, they can create psychological roadblocks or even diagnoses that can challenge your overall well-being.

The emotional dimension includes the ways that you cope, manage, and express stress. With self-care being a process of establishing healthy routines, it is vital that emotional well-being is at the forefront. If your emotional balance is off, it may be a result of the other dimensions, one or more, being impacted by habits that are not beneficial to you.

Within the dimension of emotions, you also want to find balance. It is important to understand that you don't have to be happy 100 percent of the time. There should always be an ebb and flow to your emotions. Happiness is important, but it should be balanced with anger, anxiety, guilt, and other emotions. These emotions also serve a purpose in our lives.

A healthy emotional balance means that you find strategies to manage the range of emotions, and no single emotion is omnipresent. You are never all happy or all sad for long periods of time; you are able to ebb and flow naturally and in a healthy manner. Dr. Martin Seligman, a psychologist who studies the power of happiness, explains that "the skills of becoming happy turn out to be almost entirely different from the skills of not being sad, not being anxious, or not being angry."

Seligman[7] shifted the field of psychology, which was largely focused on looking back and finding fault in the past or historical events as an explanation for emotions that are out of balance. Instead, through experiments on learned helplessness, he began to understand the power of optimism—the power of creating healthy habits that lead to protective skills that come with hope, happiness, and optimism.

Numerous studies have even shown that your smile can impact not only your current mood but your overall health. The Duchenne Smile[8] is categorized as a smile that uses the majority of your facial muscles. What scientists continue to understand is that happiness, even the degree to which and how often you smile can impact your overall health and even life longevity.

BALANCING ACT

Creating a balance of the eight dimensions of wellness means that you are able to flourish. You have created habits of mind and body which exhibit through healthy habits and beneficial behaviors. Balance means that there will be ups and downs, ebbs and flows, and highs and lows.

Imagine life is a game in which you are juggling eight balls. These balls are the eight dimensions. You are doing your best at keeping all of them in the air, but it is a struggle. One day you finally come to understand that two of the dimensions—occupational and financial—are rubber balls; if you drop them, they will bounce back. The other balls are made of glass; if you drop one of these, it will irrevocably scuffed, nicked, and perhaps even shattered. Once you truly understand the lesson of which balls are more fragile for you, you will have the beginning of balance in your life.

The most important part of balance is that nothing becomes so overwhelming; no single or group of dimensions is creating an imbalance that results in the inability to function. When that type of imbalance occurs, seeking more professional assistance may be required. Self-care is achievable when you are seeking to find an appropriate balance. There may be times or circumstances that require outside assistance or professional psychological support to gain headway toward balance. Even in finding inner wellness, seeking outside assistance is admirable.

Traumatic events may be one circumstance where its impacts are long-lasting or too impactful to cope with on your own and that is okay. That isn't to say that experiencing trauma is going to create an imbalance that you cannot overcome, but for many, trauma can significantly impact the balance of wellness.

To understand the impacts of trauma and how trauma has the potential to create lasting impacts on overall health and wellness, the Centers for Disease Control and Prevention (CDC)[9] has created tools that are based on the study of the Adverse Childhood Experiences Study (ACES),[10] originally conducted by Kaiser Permanente. The ACES assessment essentially helps to identify a score associated with the degree to which you may have been exposed to trauma. The higher the ACES score, the greater the impact.

Exposure to trauma, which is considered to be a deeply distressing or disturbing experience, can impact your overall health and even longevity. Exposure to or experiencing trauma doesn't have to create a significant imbalance; in fact, more than 60 percent of adults studied reported having an ACE score of at least one.[11] Even with adverse childhood experiences, you can find and create a dimensional wellness balance.

There are typically four reasons that you may be out of balance. The first is that you have created routines or habits that don't align well with your self-care needs. The second is that your balance is being influenced by something outside of your current control. The third is that you simply haven't taken time to understand and find your balance. And the fourth, the intent of this book, is that your self-care routine is not aligned to your needs.

If your self-care plan is not intentional and not individualized based on your needs, then the first three reasons for imbalance may be impacted. Finding balance is about identifying strategies that will increase the potency of your wellness.

With so many options for potential self-care available to you, it can be hard to know and understand what to choose and why. Sure, you can try goat yoga or axe throwing or plate smashing or even crochet bombing, but how do you know that those are going to help create stasis for your dimensions of wellness?

This is where the science of behavior analysis comes in.

SELF-CARE SYNERGY

This chapter began with the Greek word *Metanoia*. It means *the journey of changing one's mind, heart, or way of life; spiritual conversion.*

1. Reflect on a journey that you have already gone through that changed you significantly.
2. Use this writing prompt to tell a story about a personal journey: I once was a different person, and this _____ changed me.
3. Explain to a friend what you learned about the eight dimensions of wellness.
4. Practice balancing on one foot for thirty seconds. Now practice with your eyes closed. Was the act of balancing different?

NOTES

1. Ingersoll, R. M., Merrill, E., Stuckey, D., and Collins, G. (2018). Seven Trends: The Transformation of the Teaching Force – Updated October 2018. *CPRE Research Reports*. Retrieved from https://repository.upenn.edu/cpre_research reports/108.
2. https://pdkpoll.org/results.
3. https://pdkpoll.org/results.

4. https://www.samhsa.gov/.
5. An internet resource developed by Green, C. D. http://www.yorku.ca/dept/psych/classics/author.htm. Toronto, Ontario: York University. ISSN 1492-3713.
6. https://www.medicalnewstoday.com/articles/66840#1.
7. https://www.authentichappiness.sas.upenn.edu/home.
8. Coles, N. A., Larsen, J. T. and Lench, H. C. (2019) "A meta-analysis of the facial feedback literature: Effects of facial feedback on emotional experience are small and variable." *Psychological Bulletin*, 145(6), 610–651. http://dx.doi.org/10.1037/bul0000194.
9. https://www.cdc.gov/violenceprevention/childabuseandneglect/acestudy/index.html.
10. https://www.cdc.gov/violenceprevention/childabuseandneglect/acestudy/about.html.
11. https://www.cdc.gov/violenceprevention/childabuseandneglect/aces/fastfact.html.

Chapter 2

Prajna—Sanskrit

The opposite of spiritual ignorance; Direct insight into the truth.

Insights into Applied Behavior Analysis

WHAT IS APPLIED BEHAVIOR ANALYSIS?

Behavior analysis is the study and science of the behavior of living organisms. Applied behavior analysis (ABA) is the practical application of that science to the improvement of lives. Some even claim that you can save the world[1] with behavior analysis. And the science has indeed created great gains for many.

ABA has impacted the lives of thousands of children and adults with autism and cognitive disabilities. ABA has influenced the design of zoos and the treatment of animals in the entertainment industry. It is used in the training of professional and Olympic athletes. ABA has likely even influenced your school and classroom in positive ways.

CLASSICAL CONDITIONING

Classical conditioning is the process of pairing an unconditioned stimulus with a neutral stimulus so that the neutral stimulus eventually creates a conditioned response. A simple example is Pavlov's original salivating dog. The unconditioned stimulus was food. The unconditioned response was salivating when food was presented. Picture the last time that a delicious, fragrant plate of food was placed in front of you. The body's natural response is to produce saliva in order to better digest that yummy food.

The neutral stimulus is a noise, a whistle, a bell, or a clap. The food is presented, and each time a noise is presented as well. The noise is paired with the food. If the noise and the food are paired enough, the body will begin to associate the noise with the presentation of the food, and voila, soon just the sound will produce the salivation. There is no magic number for the number of times the sound has to be paired, but the science of behavior has developed some criteria of best practices that help to guide the process. In later chapters, you'll learn more about collecting data and identifying patterns to understand trends and better know when changes are being made.

Now, imagine that the delicious plate of food, the best meal ever, is paired with something unpleasant, something aversive. That process can create a fear or a phobia, much like what happened in the Little Albert experiment.[2] Little Albert was a young boy who was emotionally conditioned to fear a white rabbit. The psychologist John Watson in the early 1920s was furthering his research on conditioning and developed an experiment to better understand the development of fears and phobias.

Both of these processes of stimuli pairing occur in our lives without us taking much notice. Each day stimuli that are pleasant or unpleasant are presented, and those can impact our physiological and psychological systems. Consider a time that you ate a specific meal or food item and developed an illness soon after. Do you continue to associate that food and illness together? Do you avoid eating that food? Many people make a connection between what may be a neutral stimulus to a response. In some cases, the outcome may indeed be causal, but in some cases, the outcome could just have been paired enough times or at the right time to create an aversion, an avoidance response.

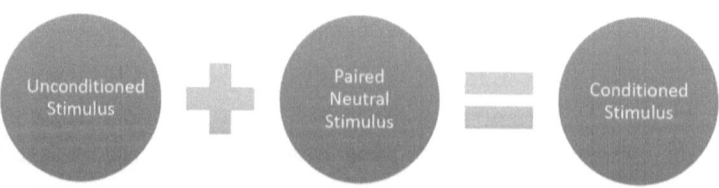

Figure 2.1 Classical Conditioning. *Source:* Author.

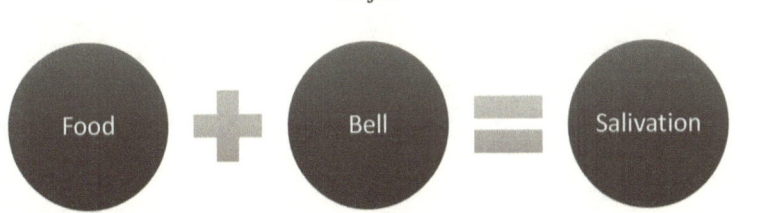

Figure 2.2 Classical Conditioning Food Example. *Source:* Author.

OPERANT CONDITIONING

B. F. Skinner built upon what Pavlov and Watson developed. He worked to further understand and develop the pairing process. Skinner was most interested in the process of responding to stimuli. He was also a creative engineer of sorts and developed a tool to help record the response of laboratory animals to different stimuli; the device is still known today as the "cumulative or event recorder."[3] If you think about your own classroom and the tools you use to monitor behaviors or chart academic gains, they are likely rooted in this rich history of behavioral theory.

Through ongoing deliberate experimentation, the process of operant conditioning was born. Operant conditioning is the process of associating specific outcomes with behaviors. The outcomes are known as reinforcement and punishment. The process works similarly to the pairing process described earlier. The primary difference is that Pavlov and Watson focused on the association of the stimuli, whereas Skinner focused on the outcomes or what behaviorists call consequences. It is through the outcomes of behaviors that Skinner began to develop his theory of learning and therefore changed the beliefs about how learning occurs and how behaviors are maintained.

The fundamental environmental conditions that impact operant conditioning are reinforcement and punishment. These are environmental stimuli that are either intentionally or incidentally introduced after behaviors. Based on the impact of reinforcement or punishment, behaviors are either increased or decreased, habits are formed, and behaviors are encouraged or discouraged. These patterns are the foundation of behavioral contingencies. And these contingencies set the stage for the formation of our habits.

These processes are further separated between respondent and operant conditioning. Respondent conditioning occurs when a response is reflexive or automatic. When you touch something hot, you automatically remove

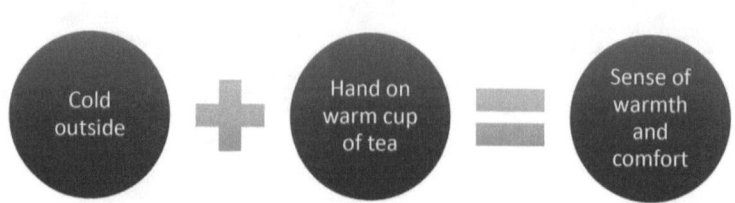

Figure 2.3 **Operant Conditioning.** *Source:* Author.

your hand from the hot stimulus. That reflex will occur whenever you touch a stimulus that is too hot.

Operant conditioning occurs when you consciously or with intent engage in a behavior. As described above, it is the consequence of that behavior that will shape the occurrence in the future. Consider when you touch that hot stimulus, but in this case, it is incredibly cold outside, and the hot stimulus is a cup of tea or coffee. The stimulus is hot and a reflexive reaction may occur initially, but the choice to hold on to the hot cup is followed by an overall warmth. The next time that it is cold outside, you may find yourself reaching for a hot cup of tea.

FORMING HABITS

Classical and operant conditioning are the foundations for how contingencies are created. Contingencies are the building blocks for our behaviors. They are the patterns that develop into habits. As described above, operant conditioning has specific outcomes that are either reinforced or punished. The outcomes of our behaviors either increase or decrease the likelihood of whether the behaviors are repeated.

In self-care, those patterns are most often referred to as habits. In many cases, we develop habits without even realizing it. Habits can be either beneficial or harmful to our everyday lives. Helpful habits might include exercising regularly or staying hydrated. They may even be habitual behaviors like preparing in advance for the week by setting out clothes or making the bed each morning.

Habits can also be or become harmful or limiting. Some habits can even develop into phobias or anxiety. Habits such as checking to see if the door is locked can be beneficial. Checking if the door is locked can become negative if it turns into a fear of the door not being locked or changing plans to ensure the door is locked and could be detrimental.

Some habits are even superstitious in nature. People begin to believe based on a repeated trend of outcomes after a behavior that a specific outcome is more likely to occur. For example, many athletes engage in habits based on superstitions. B. F. Skinner stated that "rituals are superstitions; they are adventitiously reinforced. The more conspicuous and stereotyped the behavior upon which the reinforcement is accidentally contingent, the greater the effect." For several games, they may have worn a specific pair of socks or worn their hair a certain way. If each of those games were won, they begin to attribute the winning to those behaviors, creating ongoing superstitious behaviors.

Conditioning helps us to understand how habits are developed and maintained. Remember Little Albert? In that experiment, Little Albert learned to be fearful of a white rat after it was paired with a loud noise. In operant conditioning, desired outcomes can intentionally be paired with certain behaviors to produce beneficial results. For instance, if someone wanted to increase the amount of water they drink in a day they could earn a penny for each ounce consumed in a day.

ABCS OF BEHAVIOR

In its simplest definition, behavior is everything we do. In a bit more complex manner, behavior is the response both internally and externally and both physiologically and psychologically to the environment around us. B. F. Skinner lamented that "I have to tell people that they are not responsible for their behavior. They're not creating it; they're not initiating anything. It's all found somewhere else. That's an awful lot to relinquish." Our locus of control is in our response to environmental stimuli.

What Skinner and behavior analysts have been working toward ever since is helping people to understand the relationship between the environment around and within them and the responses that result. It is sometimes referred to as a behavioral contingency or the ABCs of behavior. It is the relationship between the environment and the behavior that forms the foundation of behavior analysis.

Antecedents

"A" represents antecedent. Antecedents are the stimuli or events in the environment that occur before a behavioral response. It may be the sight of a commercial on the television that creates a need to go to the kitchen and grab a snack. It might be the announcement of a classroom activity that creates a fearful response from a student like slamming books on a desk or pouting.

Oftentimes people aren't even aware of the impetus for the behavior. Many times, a behavior appears to be "out of the blue." By applying the science of behavior, one can begin to partner the antecedent with the behavior. In most cases, an antecedent is fairly immediate to the behavioral response. For example, you see [a] commercial on television, the behavior is the physiological response of hunger and getting up to get a snack, and the consequence is that the hunger is satiated. It can feel almost subconscious. In actuality though, it follows the principles that were shared around how behaviors are conditioned or learned.

Behavior

"B" in this case stands for behavior. The behavior is the response. It is the action that occurs as a result of the antecedent. As you can imagine there is nearly an infinite amount of behaviors that occur throughout the day.

For the sake of your self-care, it will be important to focus yourself on a single behavior. This may be a behavior that has the greatest impact. This may be a behavior that occurs most frequently. It may even be a behavior that someone else is encouraging you to address. You'll work to understand and focus on a single behavior in later chapters as you develop your self-care plan. First, though, it is important to know what constitutes as behavior.

Many will argue that behavior must be observable and measurable; however, as complex human beings with large cognitive capacities, our internal thoughts also drive and are impacted by these contingencies. Many behavioral scientists commit to a strict belief that internal states or "self-talk" are not part of the contingency process. It is easy, however, to believe that the verbal behavior that occurs inside our own minds can influence external behaviors.

> According to Skinner (1974),[4] self-awareness, or self-discrimination is shaped through verbal interactions with others, thereby allowing for greater prediction and influence over an individual's own behavior. It is only when a person's private world becomes important to others that it becomes important to him. By asking questions such as "How are you feeling," for example, other members of the verbal community are, in effect, shaping an individual's ability to respond

discriminatively towards his/her own behavior. The person is "made aware of himself" by such questions and is thus in a better position to predict and control his own behavior.

How will you know what behavior to focus on? Think about your day. Close your eyes and walk through a typical day from start to finish. Consider all the items that help you to feel joyful, challenged, or uncomfortable. Do you want to focus on changing one of the harmful habits? Is there a behavior that occurs during your day that is impeding your happiness? That behavior, that habit is an area to focus on as you develop your self-care plan. This can be considered, in most cases, a limiting behavior. In this case, consider that the behavior is getting up and getting that snack. The snack is an unhealthy choice, something with saturated fats and high sodium. It can be harmful if you eat too much.

Consequences

Consequences are what happen immediately after a behavior. Consequences are not classified as either good or bad. Instead, they are the environmental responses that occur directly after the behavior. These responses can be external or can be influences from the environment around us, or they can be internal, that is, our inside story and thoughts. What is heard can influence what is thought. Those thoughts in this case become the consequences.

Consequences are what maintain behavior. They help to form the complete puzzle of what is called a contingency or the map of impact. The map of impact is a guide to help you pay more attention to the things in the environment that happen right before your challenging behavior and right after the behavior. This map will also help to determine how and when to make changes that will be more beneficial to your self-care and overall wellness.

An impact map is an opportunity to see the ABC contingency. It is the first step in your self-care expedition, much the way a map is often the starting point of a journey. Review the impact map below and practice filling one in by going to the self-care plan and completing the first section.

The greatest challenge with human behavior is just how complicated people can be. In the simple conditioning process, there is a stimulus and a response. In the contingency process, there is an antecedent, a behavior, and a consequence. In everyday life, there is so much more. In the mind, there is so much more. In the classroom, there is so much more. Behaviors are not just

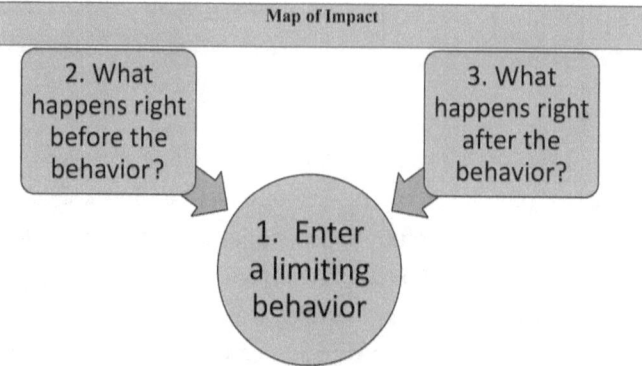

Figure 2.4 Map of Impact. *Source:* Author.

impacted by the immediate before and after in many cases; they are impacted by the outcomes of things that happened years ago in the past or thoughts of what could happen in the future.

The consequences that occur after behaviors are vital to understanding the habits that are formed. In behavioral science, consequences either reinforce or punish the behavior that occurred. Consequences either keep those behaviors going or stop the behaviors from continuing; they are neither good nor bad, just after.

REINFORCEMENT AND PUNISHMENT

Reinforcers are the consequences that occur after target behaviors and maintain or increase the likelihood that those behaviors will occur. Punishers are the consequences that occur after target behaviors and decrease or eliminate those behaviors. Again, they don't mean good or bad. Rather, they result in that the behavior happens more or happens less.

In behavioral science, there are both positive and negative influences on reinforcers and punishers. Positive means that something is added to the environment. Negative means that something is removed from the environment.

Now consider some of the harmful habits that occur on a regular basis. Perhaps it is nail-biting or negative self-talk. There are reinforcers that are maintaining those behaviors, those habits, even when they may not be healthy. If a behavior continues, there is something in the environment occurring soon after it that maintains it.

Table 2.1 Reinforcement and Punishment

Description of Reinforcement and Punishment		
	Reinforcement (+)	*Punishment (-)*
Positive (+)	Something Added	Something Added
	Behavior Increases	Behavior Decreases
Negative (-)	Something Removed	Something Removed
	Behavior Increases	Behavior Decreases

It can be hard to believe that people would continue to do things that aren't healthy, but evidence of this can be seen all over. People who eat heavily sugared or salted foods even after being diagnosed with a health concern. People who speed or text and drive even after seeing accidents or receiving costly tickets. Even people who physically harm themselves or become addicted to harmful substances.

Reinforcement of unhealthy habits can also be seen in smaller, more subtle behaviors, such as looking in the mirror and seeing perceived flaws or spending time on the weekend writing lesson plans or grading work instead of spending time with family or being outdoors. And punishment of healthy behaviors can occur without much fanfare as well. This happens when immediate results from a diet aren't seen or a medication doesn't result in pain reduction.

What is important in a self-care routine is to become more aware and conscious of the As (antecedents) and Cs (consequences) of the behavior you are trying to address. It is also important to understand the ways in which you are motivated to continue healthy and helpful habits.

Reinforcers can either be internal or external. Reinforcers that are internal are considered intrinsic. This essentially means that it is the joy of the activity alone that maintains the behavior. Intrinsic motivators are commonly associated with learning to play an instrument or sometimes even exercise. It assumes that you would engage in the activity without any external reward.

On the other hand, there are some behaviors that include some form of external reward to help with motivation. These external rewards are often referred to as extrinsic. Those behaviors aren't as easy or enjoyable, so they may need an external source of motivation. For example, learning a new skill or routine may be difficult and require an additional source of encouragement.

For instance, if you learn a new workout every day for two straight weeks, you may reward yourself with a new workout outfit or spa day.

Take a moment to think about those activities that you simply love to do. You almost lose yourself in the activity. It may be a hobby or a sport. You don't desire money as a reward. You just enjoy doing it. That is likely something that is intrinsically motivating.

Personally, I practice yoga. To be more specific, I practice hot yoga. And though it is a difficult routine at times, the benefits that I feel are more than just physical. I have been able to connect with myself on a deeper level. I have been able to learn to breathe into spaces that are stressful or uncomfortable. I have learned to connect my breath to my body and my mind. I practice yoga for a number of reasons, but mostly because I enjoy it. And I practice it in some small way every day. I slow my breath, I focus my energy, and I slow my pace. I don't need a reminder to do these activities; I do them because they are part of my life now.

Now think of those activities that you need a little more encouragement. A reward at the end is worth the effort. The reward may not be financial; it may be a goal that is met or an accomplishment that is acknowledged by someone. That is likely something that is extrinsically motivating.

I also trained to run a half marathon. I am not inherently a runner. I am not shaped like a graceful gazelle, but more like a little mouse. I ran for the challenge to prove that I could accomplish the goal; however, every run required a motivator. I would run with a friend to stay encouraged along the way. I would treat myself to ice cream after. I would buy new shoes or new running pants. I didn't run just for the sake of the enjoyment of running; I ran for a purpose, a reward.

The great thing is, through strategizing the reinforcers and punishers, you can develop intrinsic joy for those activities that initially require extrinsic rewards. Consider when you have to learn a new skill. It can be difficult at first and perhaps there is little immediate joy in the outcomes. You may even give yourself small rewards for completing steps of the learning process. At some point, you require fewer and fewer of those rewards because the learning becomes easier or the joy of accomplishment becomes greater.

While I never did gain that intrinsic "runners high" that so many proclaim exist. I did begin to enjoy the practice of being outside, being active, being part of a community of active people. Less and less along the way did I require the external rewards and at some point, the joy of being a runner took over. I then transferred that love into the practice of yoga, which also has a community feel. I accomplished the goal of completing two half marathons and now I challenge myself every time I am on my yoga mat with personal goals. I continue to successfully surpass my goals through both external and internal rewards.

You likely see this in your students as they learn new skills all the time. In the beginning they may require a lot of your attention and praise. At some point, they need less support and less encouragement. Once they've mastered a skill they likely continue to flourish and hopefully even enjoy using their new skill. It can be learning new words, math problems, even social and emotional skills. The same strategies that you apply every day in the classroom to support learning are what you are working to do for your self-care routine.

SCHEDULES OF REINFORCEMENT

Reinforcers and punishers are ultimately the list of consequences from the ABC activity. The list in column C, those environmental factors that occur directly after the behavior are what is maintaining the behavior. That means that what falls under column C is either increasing or maintaining the limiting behaviors (reinforcement) or decreasing the limiting behaviors (punishment).

Schedules of reinforcement can impact all facets of your life and routines. The timing of reinforcement and the way in which it is carried out can help to develop helpful behavior patterns or harmful behavior patterns. B. F. Skinner proclaimed that "the way in which reinforcement is carried out is more important than the amount." The more you are able to identify and recognize the power of reinforcement in your self-care routine, the stronger and deeper the benefit.

There are several schedules of reinforcement or ways in which reinforcers are delivered. Below in the figure, you can see that reinforcers are either fixed or variable. Fixed means there is consistency, and variable means there is a range. There are also two types of reinforcers: a ratio and an interval. A ratio is a number, and an interval is a measure of time that occurs.

It is not necessary to become an expert in the science of behavior, but there is necessity in paying attention to how the environment impacts your decisions and your behaviors. Skinner once stated that

Table 2.2

Schedules of Reinforcement	Ratio	Interval
Fixed	Reinforcement after a **consistent NUMBER** of responses	Reinforcement after a **consistent** amount of **TIME**
	Example: Every sip of water that you take you earn a penny	Example: Every time you drink 8 ounces of water within an hour you earn a dollar
Variable	Reinforcement after an **average NUMBER** of responses	Reinforcement after an **average** amount of **TIME**
	Example: When you drink between 5 and 10 sips of water you earn a penny	Example: When you drink 64 ounces of water while you are awake (approximately 8 hrs) you earn 50 dollars

behavior is a difficult subject matter, not because it is inaccessible, but because it is extremely complex. Since it is a process, rather than a thing, it cannot be held still for observation. It is changing, fluid, evanescent and for this reason it makes great technical demands on the ingenuity and energy of the scientist.

You are not working to become a scientist; you are working to become a *selfist*—a person focused on creating the best possible circumstances for happiness and health.

SELF-CARE SYNERGY

This chapter began with the Sanskrit term *Prajna* which means *the opposite of spiritual ignorance; Direct insight into the truth.*

1. Science is often seen as a process of discovering the truth. Create a story about something you didn't believe in but now know is true or real.
2. List three ways that you have experienced or observed reinforcement and punishment in the classroom (in your job).
3. Draw a picture of what you believe to be the powerful reinforcer you could receive.
4. Observe an animal in nature. Choose a single behavior and determine what happens right before the behavior and right after the behavior.

NOTES

1. https://dickmalott.com/.
2. https://www.apa.org/monitor/2010/01/little-albert.
3. Skinner, B. F. (1959) *Cumulative Record*. New York: Appleton Century Crofts.
4. Skinner, B. F. (1974) *About Behaviorism*. New York: Knopf.

Chapter 3

Acora Imparo—Italian

Yet, I am learning.

Wellness in the Learning Space

HABITS IN THE CLASSROOM

Our habits are essentially part of a contingency, part of a process of conditioning. In the classroom our habits also have an impact. Some people develop the habit of standing in a specific area of the classroom or following the same routine every morning. These habits could be beneficial or detrimental. Some educators develop habits of being early or late to meetings. Some people develop habits of consuming caffeine or sugar to stay energized during the day. These habits can all either help or limit.

Students in the classroom also develop habits. They develop personal and academic habits and those again can either help or harm their progress. The more that is understood about how behaviors are impacted, the better able to make necessary shifts toward improvement.

Students are also paying close attention to your behaviors and habits. Theories of social learning posit that as humans we are all also learners. We observe behaviors and patterns of behavior and through that observation we learn direct or indirect impacts. This means that as the educator in the classroom, not only are our students learning from us but we are also constantly learning.

Our students, as learners, are observing our behaviors in the classroom throughout the day. Associate Professor of Education, Patricia Jennings stated that

> "The primary way children learn social-emotional skills is through being exposed to adult behavior," said Patricia Jennings, an associate professor of education at the University of Virginia who studies teacher stress and the social and emotional context of the classroom. "If a teacher doesn't have a level of social-emotional competence to model the kinds of behaviors that he or she is hoping students adopt, then he or she is sending mixed messages."

Not only is it important for our cup to be full and our self-care "account" above the red line, but it is important that we help to teach those self-care behaviors to our students.

APPLIED BEHAVIOR ANALYSIS IN THE CLASSROOM

Applied behavior analysis (ABA) has likely influenced a number of your personal and educator processes as well. The science can be invaluable to educators who may want to create strong classroom management practices or address challenging behaviors. The roots of many common classroom strategies are derived from behavior analysis.

These common strategies that you use every day in the classroom can be applied to your self-care practices as well. Consider that what works well for you as an educator may work well for you outside of the classroom or in your personal life, if applied correctly. In the same way that you value the power of establishing routines in the classroom, you also can benefit from appropriate boundaries in your personal life as well. In the same way that you create and maintain engagement for new topics, you also can benefit from sound instructional techniques. When you develop systems to reward and recognize students, you also need that recognition.

When you begin the process of designing your self-care plan in later chapters, come back to what you know works so well for your students, in the classroom or throughout the school setting. Remember that as humans, our environment and the contingencies that are present influence us all. Spend the same level of effort, if now more, on yourself than you do to ensure your students are successful and have a high quality of life.

CLASSROOM CONNECTIONS

Many of you have likely either used or have seen a color chart as a classroom management strategy. The concept is that students move up and down a chart that displays their level of behavior. If they are behaving well, they stay at the top of the chart. If they exhibit challenging behaviors, they have to move down the chart.

There are two important things to consider with this behavioral system. One, it is public—everyone can see how everyone else is doing. This can work for some students but can also be embarrassing for some children. For students that are still learning the skills necessary to behave appropriately, it may also overinflate and emphasize a skill deficit rather than a behavioral deficit, which in turn could create an emotional deficit.

Apply the same system to your self-care. Have you ever taken a spin class or group exercise class? If you are confident with your skills, you may not mind a leader board in the front of the class announcing everyone's position. But if you are new to the class, it may feel defeating to see your name drop at the bottom of the pack. After all, you have the right motivation and interest, and you are simply still learning.

In yoga, you are instructed to not compare yourself to others. It is an important self-care lesson that the practice of yoga emphasizes. When engaging in a class practice, it is about you and what you can achieve on your mat. Some days are better than others, and some sides are stronger than others. And, that's okay. You are only in competition with the goals that you set for yourself.

Consider that color chart again. The behavioral root is sound—let an individual know immediately if their behavior is appropriate or not. The application of the practice though may not fit each individual, much the way the self-care comparisons also may or may not fit. Much the way you individualize supports for students, you'll be working on individualizing your self-care and learning what works best for you.

Another common strategy is token economies—the marble jars, sticker systems, faux money and other money-based systems that are created for the classroom. The behavioral basis and intent for token economies are to provide an immediate reinforcer for the appropriate behavior (the ticket) that can then be submitted later for a larger reward, usually a treasure box or items in a school store. Not only do token economies have a rich history in behavior analysis, but they also function in your everyday life and can work for your self-care planning. If you recall, the immediacy of reinforcement is important. The longer the wait for the reinforcer, the less powerful it is and the more opportunity to inadvertently reinforce a different or inappropriate behavior.

At some point, you may have begun a diet or lifestyle change. When you don't readily see the impact of the effort you are putting in, you may not continue with the plan. If you don't see the pounds come off quickly, you may abandon the lifestyle change. If a reinforcement system is set up, like a token economy, and you are earning toward your goal, those little steps in between may feel more impactful.

Another strategy you likely use in the classroom frequently is called the Premack Principle or grandma's law. It is called grandma's law because you've likely heard a grandma say, "If you eat your vegetables first, then you can have dessert." The behavioral application is using a more highly preferred activity to reinforce a lesser preferred activity. The Premack Principle can be essential when you are initially beginning a new process or routine because the newness may not initially be reinforcing or enjoyable. When you use a more preferred activity, as the reinforcer, it can help build up momentum for success. For example, first do the yoga class, then you get to relax in the hard-earned final resting pose of *shivasana*.

Speaking of momentum, another strategy you may use in the classroom is called behavioral momentum. When applying behavioral momentum, much like the theory of momentum in physics, you use smaller preferred tasks or activities to build up toward an activity that may not be as reinforcing. In other words, you do small chunks of something you like to build up momentum for something that may not be as enjoyable. First you grow a small herb plant in a pot in your window and then you start your raised garden bed in your yard.

For example, you may not yet be ready for a ninety-minute hot power yoga class, but you may be ready to practice deep breathing techniques, then a restorative yoga class, and then a more advanced yoga experience in your home before working your way up to the hot yoga. In the classroom, this often looks like some quick and engaging question-and-answer sessions before a larger writing activity.

In most cases, there are likely hundreds of applications of the science of behavior, the fundamentals of the stimulus-response relationship and the power of reinforcers and punishers that you use in the classroom on a regular basis. These now are going to be the same fundamental principles that you begin to apply to your self-care plan. If you consider what works best for you when you are teaching others, those are the strategies to apply when you are teaching yourself.

Researcher and policy advocate Andy Hargreaves said, "Students become good learners when they are in the classes of teachers who are good learners." Bandura's theory of social learning emphasizes this notion by acknowledging that people learn through modeling and observation. Additional education researchers talk about the value of educators having strong social and emotional competence in order to best model those skills for students.

All of these theorists and researchers are focused on the value of the educator as the primary source for helping to build an environment of social-emotional learning that includes self-care. The science of ABA is now going to be added to this foundation in order to solidify you as the center of importance. Self-care is not selfish. Self-care is one of the most selfless acts available because it will allow you to share, model, and teach your students how to create a quality of life that reflects the eight dimensions of wellness. Now it is time to connect science with self-care.

SELF-CARE SYNERGY

This chapter began with the Italian phrase *Acora Imparo*, which means y*et, I am learning.*

1. Make a list of one thing you already knew about self-care, one thing that you learned in this chapter about self-care, and one thing that you still hope to learn more about.
2. Close your eyes and picture the best day that you ever had in the classroom or at school. What made the day so special? Who was there? How did you feel? What were the sounds and smells?
3. Create a to-do list of items you can adjust in your instructional and/or classroom management practices.
4. With a family member or friend, practice using one of the behavioral strategies like behavioral momentum or the Premack Principle.

Chapter 4

Ikigai—Japanese

A reason for being.

Understanding the Reason for Being

UNDERSTANDING WHY

One of the first steps in making a change in habits or behaviors is to understand *the why*. Why you may have developed specific patterns and how those have impacted your daily life over time. B. F. Skinner said, "Education is what survives when what has been learned has been forgotten." For many years, behavior analysis has been considered a process of manipulation, removal of free will or choice. It has been seen as the simplistic process of stimulus—response. It has even been misunderstood as a process of merely rewarding external behaviors.

B. F. Skinner, however, hoped that it would become a science to change the world. Many of his writings focused on how science could be applied to understanding human behavior, improving organizations and industries, and most importantly, impacting the field of education. What survives after what has been learned is forgotten are those behaviors that have become habits, those actions that are ingrained, lasting, and ongoing. The goal of the science of behavior analysis is to begin to understand *why* those behaviors continue, and what maintains those behaviors to increase the quality of life of individuals or groups.

Have you ever had a student or group of students in your class that have exhibited challenging or disruptive behaviors? Have you ever felt at a loss because a student's behavior was limiting their potential or impacting the learning of others? Perhaps you've experienced the difficulty that a particular child brings to the classroom. Consider the story of Maurice.

Maurice was just beginning middle school. This school was the ninth school that Maurice had attended. Maurice lived with his single mother who was in and out of abusive relationships, back and forth with law enforcement, and up and down with illicit drug use. Maurice spent a great deal of time with his caring but inattentive grandparents.

His behavior was mostly internal; he spent his time in his own mind. Yet, his behavior was explosive. Most teachers would likely say that his aggression "came out of nowhere."

In the world of behavior analysis, there is always an underlying cause, a reason for the explosion. Our job, the job of the teacher and school support staff, is to understand the why. Why was Maurice so angry?

Maurice was volatile. He was explosive at times. In many homes in wintery regions, typically in the dark and dank basement is a large antiquated dinosaur-like appliance. Anyone who knows this appliance knows that they require attention. A furnace if left unattended can literally explode.

Every so often, the homeowner, in an attempt to maintain the furnace, is required to trek to the basement and carefully twist the valve on the machine. This process releases pent-up steam and allows the furnace to function, to breathe, and to continue to work. Maurice was that furnace. This may feel like the same built-up stress that you feel when new curriculum, new demands, new expectations, or new students place on your routine.

The best way to reduce the risk of emotional explosions is to begin to understand the why. In some instances, you may have even felt those emotional explosions. In behavior analysis, the why is the function of the behavior. The function of the behavior helps to determine why a behavior is occurring which will then help to develop an improvement plan.

FUNCTIONS OF BEHAVIOR

Behavior is anything that we say or do. Behavior is everything that we say and do. The functions of behavior are the reasons why we say and do what we say and do.

There are traditionally four functions of behavior, four ways to get or get away from people or things, and four main reasons why behavior occurs. They are easy to remember by using the acronym, SEAT—Sensory, Escape/Avoidance, Attention, and Tangible. Understanding the function of any behavior is the first step in developing a plan for the best quality of life.

Sensory

Sensory is a function of behavior that is less common in most classrooms but is directly connected to self-care. Most people engage in sensory behavior simply because it feels good—the way that listening to music or curling up in a soft blanket may feel. The distinguishing feature from other functions, however, is that sensory behaviors will occur in the absence of anyone else. A person will engage in sensory behaviors if nothing and no one is around.

If you have ever tried to ignore an itch, you know the power of sensory as function of behavior. Sensory behaviors are most often associated with the

Sensory	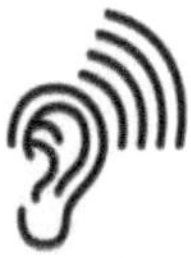 👂
Escape/Avoidance	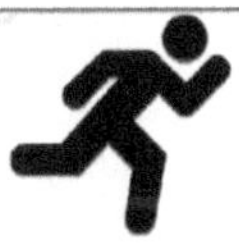 🏃
Attention	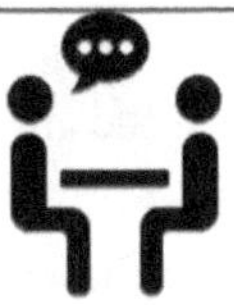 💬👥
Tangible	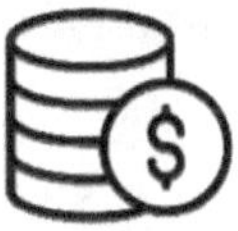 💰

Figure 4.1 Functions of Behavior. *Source*: Author.

pleasure center of the brain. Sensory behaviors are aligned directly to the five senses: smelling, tasting, hearing, seeing, and touching or feeling. Sensory behaviors can occur at any time and are likely to be associated with a physiological component.

Escape/Avoidance

With behavior we are either trying to get something or get away from something. With escape and avoidance, it is a desire to get away from people or things. Escape and avoidance behaviors can occur to remove something unpleasant or remove yourself from something unpleasant.

Escape and avoidance are slightly different. Escape means that you are already engaged in the activity or with the person and you escaping the undesired stimulus. Avoidance means that you anticipate something unpleasant and work to avoid the circumstance, like the work acquaintance who you actively avoid because you know she will only complain or vent at you and never allow you the time to vent or having to go to an event where you won't know anyone.

It is common to experience escape and avoidance and especially to see these functions in the classroom. Have you ever had a student who would melt down before a difficult task or subject? Or have you ever arrived early or left late from school to avoid an unfriendly colleague?

Escape and avoidance are appropriate in some cases. They build on our innate survival skills but if you continue to avoid harmless situations or escape from every activity, it can be detrimental. In self-care, you can learn how to use escape and avoidance to your advantage.

Attention

Attention is probably the most common function of behavior. Humans are social creatures. It is normal for people to want to interact with other people and for people to want the attention of other people.

In the classroom, you've likely seen attention as a function manifest as the student who calls out in class or is always at your desk with a question. As adults it can be the person who is always the loudest in the room or has to have the spotlight in a meeting. Attention is all about getting a response from another person. In some cases, people even want negative or bad attention because they are hungry for any form of attention. You may have witnessed this with kids in the classroom who will act out even if they are reprimanded. Think of it like this: when you are starving, even bad food can taste good.

Tangible

The function of tangible is related to things and activities. When someone engages in a behavior with the function of tangible, they are trying to access a preferred activity or item. You'll see behaviors that are related to the function tangible when a child asks for a toy or when they take one away from another child. As an adult, tangible may look like the person who always wants the account login for your streaming service.

WORKING TOGETHER

All four of the functions of behavior can either work for a person or against them. The goal is to understand the why, the function, to best plan for how to ensure the behavior works for you. In self-care there has been a focus on the eight dimensions of wellness without the understanding of why self-care behaviors may be working for you or may be hindering progress.

Psychiatrist Viktor Frankl said, "Between stimulus and response is a space. In that space is our power to choose our response. In our response lies our growth and our freedom." This is the blend of behavior analysis and self-care. That space and that choice are built on the foundation of the functions of behavior and the way in which they influence the eight dimensions of wellness.

By learning about and understanding why you engage in certain behaviors, by investigating your routines and paying attention to your habits, you will be better able to identify the dimensions of wellness that will best suit you or the ones that require your focus. By understanding the why you can grow.

As author Brianna Weist states, self-care is more than just establishing a new healthy routine.

> It means being the hero of your life, not the victim. It means rewiring what you have until your everyday life isn't something you need therapy to recover from. It is no longer choosing a life that looks good over a life that feels good. It is giving the hell up on some goals so you can care about others. It is being honest

even if that means you aren't universally liked. It is meeting your own needs so you aren't anxious and dependent on other people.

It is becoming the person you know you want and are meant to be. Someone who knows that salt baths and chocolate cake are ways to enjoy life—not escape from it.

In order to do this, you have to take a deeper look at yourself. You have to be honest with yourself and vulnerable. You have to focus on you. Observe your interactions, your thoughts, and your inner dialogue.

The best way to do this is to assess yourself, in the same way that you would observe and assess a student that was struggling with an academic subject or who exhibits challenging behavior. You may not yet know or see how your behavior is affecting you or your success on the self-care journey.

In behavior analysis the traditional method is a functional behavioral assessment. This is a process of defining target behaviors, observing and collecting data, responding to self-reflection questions, and developing a hypothesis of the function of behavior, the why.

In the next chapters, you will engage in a similar process. To help develop your self-care plan, you'll be engaging in the four-dimensional (4-D) planning process to discover, define, design, and do the self-care activities that will offer you the greatest benefit.

SELF-CARE SYNERGY

This chapter began with the Japanese term *Ikigai*, meaning a *reason for being*.

1. As part of a lesson plan or activity in the classroom or with a student, ask them to describe their reason for being.
2. Draw a picture of your best day. What were sensory components (sights, smells, etc.) in the scenario? Who or what were you surrounded by? What worries or stressors did you forget all about because of how wonderful the day was? Who were the conversations, what made you smile or laugh?
3. Experience a guided meditation of Maurice and the furnace:
    a. Sit somewhere where you can be quiet and free from distraction for several minutes.

b. Close your eyes and take several deep breaths.
c. Imagine Maurice. Picture all of the details of his face, his clothing, and his mannerisms.
d. Watch him begin to get upset and frustrated. Observe his body language.
e. Let him know that it is time to release the steam and cool off.
f. Picture a small valve being turned and steam releasing from Maurice's ears.
g. Watch as he calms.
h. Take a few deep breaths.
i. Feel that same sense of calm.
j. Open your eyes.
4. Write down everything that you do for one day and reflect on how many behaviors we engage in each and every day.

Chapter 5

Amat Victoria Curam—Latin

Victory loves preparation.

Planning and Preparation for Self-Care

PLANNING FOR SELF-CARE

It may seem counterintuitive or strange to talk about planning for self-care. It's likely something that should occur based on need or under certain circumstances, but much like your overall physical health, it's beneficial to establish a wellness routine. Consider if you went in to each day of teaching with no plan at all!

It is especially important to revisit when you identify something in your current routine or wellness plan that isn't working. You may not have a balance in the eight dimensions of wellness or you've established some unhealthy routines because you haven't addressed the function of behaviors inhibiting healthy choices. Also, you may just be interested in establishing new habits that help you feel better.

No matter the reason, the best place to start is the same place you begin any problem-solving process, by understanding what is and is not working: in this case, *discovering* your healthy and not-so healthy habits. You'll continue on your journey by first *defining* the self-care behaviors that you want *or need* to target. Next, you'll begin *designing* a plan matching the dimensions of wellness you want to target aligned with the functions of behavior. Finally, you'll *do* the plan, which means you'll put it into action.

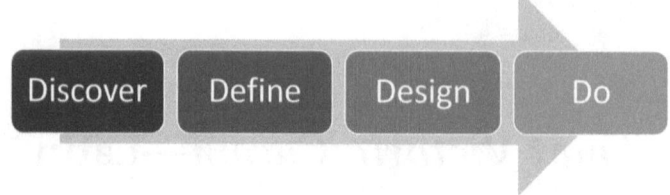

Figure 5.1 Four-Part Problem-Solving Process. *Source*: Author.

DISCOVER

Discovery is a process of searching for something. Discovery is also about finding something. Like following the X on a treasure map to search and find a treasure, discovery is about unlocking potential and locating the path toward a goal.

> *Discovery consists of looking at the same thing as everyone else and thinking something different.*
>
> Albert Szent-Gyorgyi

You are going to begin the discovery phase by reflecting on your habits and routines, what is the pattern of your day, and what works and doesn't work. In earlier chapters, you took some time to think about it and reflect. Now is the time to dig deeper and document the process.

Discovery is about understanding "what first" so that you will be better prepared to understand the "why." In order to do this, you'll complete the first section of your self-care plan below and begin the Four D process of developing your self-care plan. If you need to spend a day or two paying closer attention to your habit and routines, observe yourself with grace and then sit down to complete Section One of the self-care plan.

Great work on starting your plan! Did you learn anything new about yourself that surprises you? Were you able to observe your habits and routines in a way that led to additional self-discovery?

In the process of discovery, you have learned that you have habits or limiting behaviors that are impacting your happiness. You may have discovered that your thoughts do not align with what is happening around you. You may have discovered that there are people in your life who are not championing your success. On your self-care journey, you do not need to make sweeping

Table 5.1 Section One: Self-Care Plan

	Section One: Discover	
Why are you investing in yourself?		
How will investing in yourself help you as an educator?		
List three *harmful* habits that you currently have.	1. 2. 3.	
List three *healthy/helpful* habits that you currently have.	1. 2. 3.	
What are some ways to increase your healthy/helpful habits?		
List any strategies you have tried or considered in the past or new ideas that you'd like to try.		
Write down the typical pattern of your day Morning Afternoon Evening		
During your day, what are the people, places, items, or activities that *don't* bring you much happiness?		
List three people that bring you joy.	1. 2. 3.	
List three places that bring you joy.	1. 2. 3.	
List three items that bring you joy.	1. 2. 3.	
List three activities that bring you joy.	1. 2. 3.	

changes right away; you simply have to be cognizant and willing to make some adjustments. You want to be prepared to invest in yourself.

You certainly don't have to have all the answers now. You can always go back and tweak your plan based on new observations. Self-care plans, just like most plans, are fluid and agile. The goal is just to pay a little more attention to those behaviors that are having an impact on your wellness. This will become clearer as you begin the next phase of the Four D process, defining the behavior.

SELF-CARE SYNERGY

This chapter started with the Latin phrase *Amat Victoria Curam*, which means *victory loves preparation.*

1. Tell a colleague about a day that you felt unprepared in the classroom. What did it feel like? What did you do? What was the outcome?
2. Go on a scavenger hunt or play I-spy. What were you able to discover while playing the game?
3. Call all three people on your list that bring you joy and let them know that you appreciate them.
4. Write a fun story about the three items that bring you joy. Use this writing prompt: If I had a billion dollars, I would still own these three items because _____.

Chapter 6

Kujichagulia—African

To define ourselves, name ourselves, create for ourselves and speak for ourselves.

Creating and Defining Self-Care

DEFINE

Next, you'll be developing a definition of a limiting behavior or behaviors that aren't serving you well. These are those behaviors that when you reflected in the discovery phase, you realized were not enjoyable or in some cases may be harmful. This is the routine that doesn't have a positive benefit of the activity that doesn't help you feel better.

It may not seem important to define this behavior or set of limiting behaviors, but defining limiting behaviors allows you to have the opportunity to observe, track, and better understand when and how the behavior occurs. In order to define the limiting behavior, it will require you to pay closer attention to it. This will help you to determine the *why* or the function of that behavior, thereby helping to create a more aligned self-care plan.

Remember the map of impact that you drafted? That was your first step in the process of defining the behaviors that will drive the self-care plan. Throughout the definition process, you'll build on that initial map and create a more comprehensive definition.

Think back or look back to the three harmful habits you listed in Part One of the self-care plan. Take a moment, close your eyes. What is it about those behaviors that seem to decrease your happiness or joy? Is it something that happens before or after you engage in the behavior? Is it a lack of feeling rewarded after the behavior?

For example, if a harmful behavior is overeating or shopping too frequently, is there something about how you feel right before or right after that behavior that is depleting the enjoyment or reducing the balance of other dimensions of wellness? Have you ever paid attention to what happens before and after the limiting behavior? If you have ever experienced emotional or stress eating and you eat too much, you may feel emotionally guilty and physically bloated or in pain. If you shop too frequently, you feel a sense of excitement before shopping and a sense of guilt or dissatisfaction after. In both cases, it is important to know what happened before and after the limiting behavior.

In behavior analysis, the antecedent and the consequence are fundamental to the contingency. What happens right before and right after a behavior is incredibly important; they tell the story that helps determine the *why*, the function. In the next section of the self-care plan, you are going to formally monitor and observe in order to track a limiting behavior for a period of time to understand what happens right before and right after. For now, only pick one behavior, as it's easier to track that way. Once you are proficient with monitoring and tracking, you can begin to observe additional behaviors.

In order to pick the right limiting behavior to track, consider the following: Is the behavior happening frequently, is the behavior having a significant impact, or is it impacting the normal functioning of your day? When choosing a limiting behavior to focus on, first, there are two schools of thought: one is to choose the behavior that is having the greatest impact on your life, and the second is to choose the behavior that you can most quickly see a change in. Either of the two is perfectly fine. Remember that this process is all about improving the overall quality of life, so feel free to choose the behavior that you are most comfortable addressing.

After identifying the behavior, the next step is working on defining the behavior. In behavior analysis, it is called an operational definition. It is a detailed definition of the behavior that includes several components. You want to define the behavior in a way that is observable and measurable. In other words, it can be seen, observed, and counted.

One way to test your definition is to use the potato test. If a potato can do it, then it probably isn't a behavior. In self-care there are a lot of internal behaviors, emotions, feelings, and so on. For your definition, you'll want to consider how to define it in a way that you can easily track it. If it is an emotion, are there behaviors that accompany it (i.e., anxiety nail-biting, shortness of breath, face feeling flushed)? If it is a feeling, is there a consistent internal dialogue that happens (i.e., negative self-talk, e.g., "I can't do this" or "this is too hard")?

An operational definition also often has a description of the topography of behavior. The topography describes what the behavior looks like and or sounds like. Like the bumps on a map, the topography helps to describe exactly what is happening. It may include details like how often, how much, how big or small, and how hard or soft.

A quality definition of your limiting behavior will be so clear that if you wrote it down and handed it to a stranger, they'd be able to track the behavior and report back how often or how long the behavior occurred. Again, this may be a bit more difficult with some of the less obvious behaviors, but see some of the examples below for help or ideas.

Once you are comfortable with a behavior to begin tracking, you'll start observing. You'll be paying attention and tracking what happens before and after that behavior. Remember that the antecedent is what happens before a behavior, and the consequence is what happens after the behavior. These are not positive or negative impacts, but simply observations of what occurs. The best and most effective way to track the A's (antecedents) and C's (consequences) is the use a T-chart. You'll be completing the data collection using the chart in the self-care plan below, but in a pinch you can find any blank piece of paper and create three columns, A, B, and C.

Now that you've tracked the A's ad C's for a week, what do you observe? Is there a pattern or a trend in what happens before and/or after the limiting behavior? What is that pattern? Do you get compliments on new items? Do you reduce hunger after eating? Do you connect with new people or find new information while scrolling on social media? These consequences may not be inherently bad or wrong, but they may be impacting your overall health and wellbeing in a way that you want to change or modify. Remember that self-care is about developing a balance that helps to create the best quality of life.

Pay attention to the C column. The pattern in this column is going to help you define the function of the limiting behavior. If you don't see a pattern yet, keep tracking in the same manner. Some patterns aren't quickly identified. Some patterns take longer to see. There is no pre-determined amount of

Table 6.1 Limiting Behaviors

Limiting Behavior	Example Definition
Overeating	Consuming an amount of food and calories that is in excess of the energy needed. Consuming an excess of food that is overtly sugary, high in calories, fatty, etc. Eating as a result of boredom, anxiety, stress, etc.
Spending too much money	Spending money that is above and beyond the financial ability or limit of the person spending. Utilizing credit for which repayment is only available at a minimum monthly payment or without repayment.
Limiting exercise	Reducing or removing any opportunities to physically move the body more than required through regular/normal daily practice.
Sleeping too little	Intentionally or unintentionally reducing sleep to the point that the body is unable to physically recover or cognitive difficulties result.
Watching television too often	Focusing on a television or electronic device, typically while sitting, having reducing physical movement, for periods of time that are in excess of 4 hours per day or watching 3 episodes of a television show consecutively without a break.
Working long hours	Focusing on or working on work-related activities beyond the scope of the required hours of employment. Working in excess of 20 hours for part-time employees or 40 hours for full-time employees without compensation. Reducing opportunities for personal activities as a result of engaging in work-related activities.
Limiting interactions with friends or family	Reducing or removing any opportunities to engage in social activities either face to face and/or virtually with people known as friends or family.
Feeling anxious	Experiencing physiological expressions of worry, fear, and nervousness, which may express as negative internal narratives, increased or rapid heart rate, increased sweating, fidgeting or restlessness of the appendages, inability to take deep breaths, etc. Vocalizing a state of unease and/or statements related to imminent negative events.

Table 6.2 Order and names of tables: Limiting Behaviors Section Two Operational Definition Section Two ABC Chart Section Two Data Collection

Section Two: Define
Write the operational definition for the limiting behavior you are going to monitor.
Create an ABC chart for one week.
Choose a *single* behavior, list, and write it in the "B" column. All week, track what happens right before ("A" column) and right after ("B" column) that behavior.
A   B   C   *e.g., too much screen time*
What trends or patterns do you notice in the "C" (consequence) column?

observation. You typically want to pay attention to the A's and C's; until you are confident you have a pattern, the same or similar thing happens after the limiting behavior. For some behaviors, this occurs quickly, while for some, it takes a bit longer.

Another tool to help you define the function of the limiting behavior is additional data monitoring. Think about what happens when you begin many new routines, you track data. If you want to swim more laps or increase the pace of running, you track your times. If you want to increase the steps you take per day, you use a tool to know how many you currently take and you likely set a goal for how many you want to take. If you begin a diet or changing your eating habits, you likely monitor calorie intake or adjust your food intake. Those are all data.

Data don't have to be intimidating or complicated. In fact, collecting data should be easy and enjoyable. These will be essential to helping you maintain your self-care change. First, you want to collect baseline data. Baseline data is a number of the current status of the behavior.

There are different kinds of data you can collect and different ways to collect it. Most commonly used is frequency. This is simply how often something happens. It's a count of how many. It can be as easy as tallying the number of times something occurs. Frequency is best used for behaviors that have a clear start and finish and for behaviors that occur quickly. For example, if a limiting behavior is internal negative statements, you would track each time you notice yourself saying something negative to yourself. Each statement has a beginning and an end, and could be counted.

Duration is another method. This tracks how long something occurs. This is good for behaviors that don't have a clear start and finish or that have multiple behaviors that occur in a cluster or together. Duration is a measurement of time, so these are often behaviors that take longer to occur or complete. An example of a limiting behavior that might use duration could be screen time or binging television/movies. While there is a stop and an end, the limiting behavior often lasts for longer periods of time and be better suited for the duration.

Another often-used data tracking system is latency. This is measured as the time between when an instruction or directive is given and the time the behavior begins. For example, if the yoga or spin instructor says to begin an exercise, latency would be the amount of time it takes you to start.

Based on the limiting behavior you are focusing on, determine which data collection method makes the most sense. Now, you'll be spending some time collecting data. There are even tools that you can use to help. You can use the timer on your phone or watch, or you can use a calorie or health app on your mobile device. There are also data collection sheets that you can download online to help you track behaviors. The self-care plan below will give you some ideas to help get you started.

Similar to ABC observations, you want to track the behaviors using the data collection method until you are able to identify a pattern. Most often, the easiest way to do this is to visualize the data or make a graphic display of the data. In other words, it's time to graph!

Again, graphing the data should be as easy as tracking it. In some cases, if you are using an online tool or an application/app, it may already provide you with a line or bar graph to help you make decisions. It is easier to identify the patterns when you can see them. Does the behavior happen most often on Tuesdays or in the mornings? Does the length of time increase in the evening or after a specific event?

Table 6.3

	Section Two: Define							
Frequency		M	T	W	Th	F	S	Su
(e.g., III II III)	6–9 am							
	9–12 pm							
	12–3 pm							
	3–6 pm							
	6–9 pm							
	9–12 pm							
	12–3 am							
	3–1 am							
Duration	Start time: _____ Stop time:_____							
(e.g., 3 pm–4:32 pm)	Start time: _____ Stop time:_____							
	Start time: _____ Stop time:_____							
	Start time: _____ Stop time:_____							
	Start time: _____ Stop time:_____							
	Start time: _____ Stop time:_____							
	Start time: _____ Stop time:_____							
	Start time: _____ Stop time:_____							
Latency	Time Instruction Given			Time Behavior Begins				
(e.g., 1:24–1:33)								

Patterns are usually considered when three or more data points continue in an upward or downward trend. For example, if you are tracking how much television you watch, the data pattern may go upward in the evenings after work and on the weekends. The length of time may increase when you have additional free time available. Another example may be that you spend less time writing in your journal on weekends or have fewer entries during times of stress. You'd be able to see these patterns on a graph

You can see in the example above of a frequency count graphed that there are some patterns that become visible about the number of times that someone says statements to themselves that are not positive. In this simple graph, you can see that on Mondays and Thursdays, the behavior occurs more often. On Sundays, it occurs the least. Depending on the behavior that is being monitored, this may help to answer some important questions about how to infuse self-care. You can also see that the behavior occurs more often toward mid-morning when looking at half of a day. If this is a limiting behavior and you are working to reduce of often it occurs, perhaps embedding some additional self-care activities on Mondays and Thursdays either just before mid-morning and right around 10:00 or 11:00 a.m. will help to create a better balance throughout the week.

Now, let's look at the same graph but view it as the duration of binge-watching TV. Now the data points represent how long a behavior lasts. The pattern may be the same in this example: Mondays and Thursdays around mid-morning are when the limiting behavior occurs most often. The time that the behavior lasts is now the focus. So, in this example, the behavior lasts the longest during that 11–12 timeframe. Perhaps the limiting behavior is negative self-talk and that timeframe is when work meetings occur. By viewing the data, you can better connect the behavior pattern to some hypothesis of why it may be occurring more often or for longer periods of time during the day.

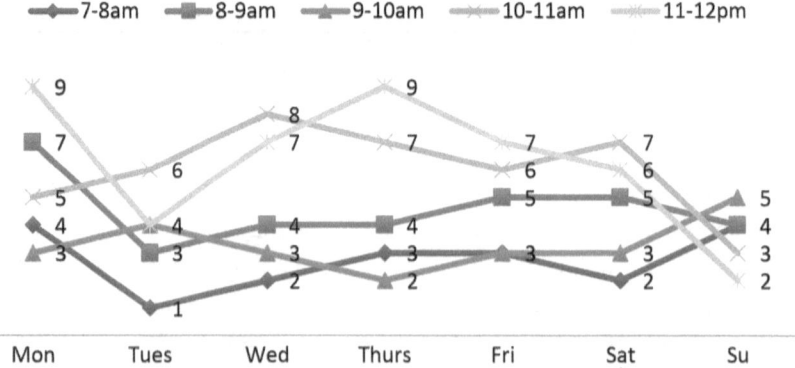

Figure 6.1 Frequency Example.

Whether you are creating the graph yourself using a graphing tool or an application that already has built-in graphs, the goal of visually displaying data is to be able to quickly view those trends and patterns. The easier it is to see what is happening, the more you'll start to make connections. The more connections you make to the behavior patterns, the closer you'll be to a strong hypothesis as to why.

The next and final step in understanding limiting behaviors and before you can begin designing your plan is to create a hypothesis of the function. The function of the behavior is the why. You have spent time now reflecting on your behavior, your habits, and your routines. You have defined a limiting behavior that is your starting place to making improvements in your overall self-care, and you've monitored that behavior to have a better understanding about why it might be occurring. Now it is time for the culmination of that work.

This process requires some analysis and synthesis. It will require you to be honest and thoughtful about the behavior and with yourself. Understanding why a behavior is occurring is *not a judgment*, but it is an answer. It is a step to finding balance.

Also, a hypothesis of the function is just that—a hypothesis. Your journey to self-care is not a single effort; it is a process—one that will likely require tweaking and adjusting. Finding balance is often ongoing. You will have the tools through this process to be more thoughtful and intentional about your self-care efforts.

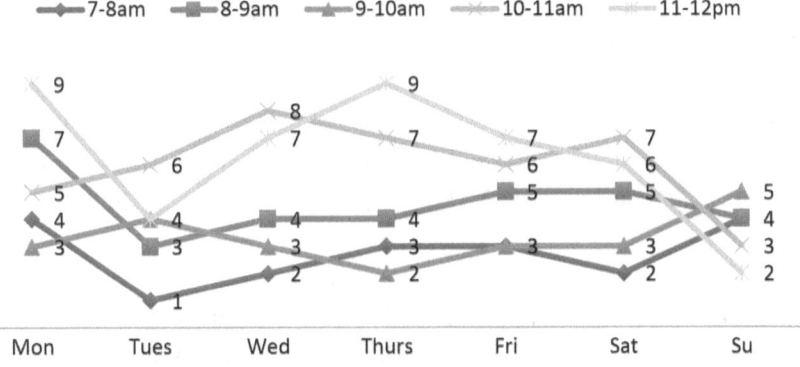

Figure 6.2 Duration Example.

Take some time to go through your entire self-care plan to this point. Review all the information that you've written down, tracked, monitored, graphed, thought about, and paid closer attention to. These are clues to your planning.

Before you create your hypothesis, here is a quick reminder about the possible functions of behavior. There are four common functions of behavior. They all result in *either gaining or getting away* from something or someone. They create the acronym SEAT.

- Sensory
- Escape/Avoidance
- Attention
- Tangible

Your hypothesis statement should look something like this:

When there is an increased workload at the office, I will sleep fewer hours at night in order to gain tangible access to "think time" to process project requirements.

When there is an increased workload at the office, I will sleep fewer hours at night in order to avoid disappointing my boss with a late or unfinished project.

When I have not seen a friend or family member in over a week, I will spend an extra 2–3 hours per day on the phone in order to gain access to attention from a family member or friend.

When I feel nervous (increased muscle movements, tight facial muscles, and clenched jaw), I will listen to loud music and can upset the neighbors, in order to gain access to sensory stimulation.

When I have to be exposed to large groups of people that I don't know well, I will remove myself from the situation and make excuses to leave in order to escape unfamiliar groups of people.

It's okay if your hypothesis isn't perfect yet. Again, give yourself grace at the beginning of this new process. You can continue to collect data. You can collect different types of data, perhaps interviewing or asking friends or family why they believe you may engage in the limiting behavior, which may

Table 6.4

Section Two: Define
Respond to the questions below.

Overview
1. What is my current limiting behavior?
2. When does it occur most often?
3. How long does it typically last?
4. What is the outcome of the limiting behavior?

Antecedents
1. What was the most commonly occurring antecedent when collecting ABC data?
2. What does that commonly occurring antecedent help me to understand about the limiting behavior?

Consequences
1. What was the most commonly occurring consequence when collecting ABC data?
2. What does that commonly occurring consequence help me to understand about the limiting behavior?
3. Is the consequence most often a person or interaction with a person?
4. Is the consequence most often getting away from someone or something?
5. Is the consequence typically gaining an item or object?

Data Collection
1. The data collection helped me realize the behavior occurs frequently.
2. The data collection helped me realize the behavior occurs for periods of time.
3. The data collection helped me realize the behavior occurs in this pattern.

Table 6.5

	Section Two: Define
Hypothesis statement for the limiting behavior	When (describe the common setting/location or environmental factors that the behavior occurs in) _____ I will (write in the limiting behavior) _____ in order to gain (add the *ONE most likely* function based on your data collection and the questions you answered above)
	Attention ☒
	Escape/Avoid ☒
	Tangible ☒
	Sensory ☒

produce some helpful information. The goal is to have a better sense of why you do what you do so that you will be more prepared to design your self-care plan and best meet your personal needs toward a wellness balance.

SELF-CARE SYNERGY

This chapter began with the African phrase *Kujichagulia*. This phrase suggests that we *define ourselves, name ourselves, create for ourselves, and speak for ourselves.*

1. Create a dictionary definition to describe you. Write your name. Spell it out phonetically. Are you a noun, a verb, an adjective? Now write your self-definition as though it would appear in a dictionary.
2. Track a positive or healthy behavior for a day. Find the antecedents and consequences for that healthy behavior. What is different from the limiting behavior? Why do you believe there is a difference?
3. Take a walk or spend time in your backyard. Look for patterns in nature. Where did you see patterns? What did the patterns look like? Why do you believe nature makes patterns?
4. Explain to a friend a time that you felt emotional (happy, sad, frustrated, joyous, etc.). Tell them in detail what the physical behaviors that accompanied the emotions. Let them know that you are paying more attention to how things inside you impact the world around you.

Chapter 7

Eunoia—Greek

A pure and well-balanced mind, a good spirit. Beautiful thinking.

Designing a Well-Balanced Self-Care Plan

DESIGN

Now that you've got the hypothesis for the function of the limiting behavior you've chosen to focus on, it's time to begin determining how you can meet that function through the dimensions of wellness. It's time to connect the eight dimensions of wellness to the four functions of behavior or, in your case, just one function of behavior for now.

Doing a simple Google search for the term "self-care activity" results in over two billion—that's correct, *billion*—results. It's no wonder that you may want to pinpoint strategies that will work best for you. You may have even tried some fraction of all those opportunities available.

As a reminder, there are eight dimensions of wellness defined by SAMHSA. Those eight dimensions create a wheel of overall holistic health. Your approach is to develop a stasis of those dimensions—a level of balance. In order to find or maintain that balance, you reflected on some behaviors that are potentially limiting your balance. You then analyzed a limiting behavior and developed a hypothesis of the why, the function, what is maintaining that limiting behavior.

Now is your opportunity to create a library of possible self-care activities that best match the function of that behavior. Now you'll be able to hone in on the specific activities that will best meet your needs. Rather than filtering through millions of options, you'll learn how to find the right kinds of activities for the purpose of finding your balance. This won't be an exhaustive list, but it should be enough to help you create your self-care toolbox. Read through each function even if it is not your focus function for the current limiting behavior; there may be a time when the function or activity will fit your needs.

SENSORY ACTIVITIES

Recall that sensory as a function will provide access or removal of stimulation to your senses. When you think of sensory as a function, think about the five senses of touch, smell, sight, feeling, and hearing. Sensory as a function for self-care activities should directly impact and influence your physical senses.

While many self-care activities may impact the senses, if sensory is the function you are focused on, you'll want your activities to specifically address the senses. For example, exercise probably sounds like a simple activity to engage in since it involves your major muscle groups. Exercise is really a healthy activity for everyone to engage in. For your personalized and function-based plan, however, you may want to be more targeted.

The following are a few examples with instructions.

Mindfulness and the Raisin

Mindfulness is a concept of grounding your thoughts to the present moment. Mindfulness can help to reduce anxiety and decrease worry since both of those emotions are influenced by past or future events. The practice of focusing on only the current moment can benefit several sensory sensations.

To begin practicing mindfulness, you'll need a raisin. Yes, just one little raisin. You can eat the rest of the healthy snack once your mindful practice is complete. Find a quiet location where you will be free from distraction or interruption for five minutes.

1. Sit comfortably.
2. Close your eyes.
3. Take slow deep breaths throughout the session.
4. Feel the weight of the raisin in your hand.

5. Roll the raisin in your palm.
6. Feel the sensation of the raisin on your hand.
7. Place the raisin close to your nose and smell.
8. Touch the raisin to your lips.
9. Feel the sensation of the raisin on your lips—is it warm, is it soft?
10. Place the raisin in your mouth.
11. Feel the weight of the raisin in your mouth.
12. Feel the texture of the raisin in your mouth.
13. Roll the raisin along your gums and along the roof of your mouth.
14. Pay attention to each sensation that you feel.
15. Feel free to eat the raisin or remove it from your mouth and discard it.
16. Write down three specific sensations that you noticed most while practicing.

It may not have seemed like much while you were practicing, but for five minutes or so, you were focused on the senses of feeling and touching, smelling, and tasting. For five minutes, you were focused on the moment. You were enveloped in sensation, and you were grounded.

Mindfulness is a sensory practice that you could engage in at any moment. You can use an item that is nearby to touch and feel. You could use the food you have for lunch, even on a busy day, to carefully focus for a few moments on the senses. If sensory is a function of your limiting behavior, consider how you could incorporate this type of sensory mindfulness practice into your daily life.

The Heart of Music

In addition to mindfulness, sensory also involves your hearing, that is, your auditory senses. To address the sense of hearing, many people turn to music. You may not realize there is music that is made for self-care. Sure, you've probably heard gentle spa music with whales and crashing waves, but there is often more going on than you realize.

There is a specific musical cadence that can directly impact your heart rate and create a calming sensation. The resting human heart beats at approximately sixty beats per second. When you become stressed, agitated, or hypervigilant, your heartbeat often elevates. Your body can go into a fight, flight, or freeze response, and prolonged episodes of elevated heart rates can impact your overall physical health.

There is music made just to soothe your ears and your heart. To practice the self-care strategy of calming music, you'll want to try the following.

1. You'll need to do a little internet searching first. Go to YouTube or any other preferred video streaming service. Use the keywords "sixty beats per minute" to search for compiled music or playlists. You may find that many classical musical compositions follow this beats per minute cadence.
2. During your first-time listening, you may want to find a quiet, distraction-free area and sit comfortably.
3. Using a music-playing device (phone, computer, laptop, tablet, etc.), play the music.
4. Take deep breaths in through your nose and out of your mouth.
5. Listen to music for at least two to five minutes.
6. When you have finished listening, write down three things that you noticed while you were listening.

Now that you know how to access the music and what to look for and listen to when you may be feeling agitated or be engaging in your limiting behavior, consider pulling up music that is sixty beats per minute to help calm and relax. This musical cadence not only addresses the sensory stimulation of hearing but also helps to train your body to calm and reduce rapid heartbeat, which can have overall health benefits, further helping to balance your wellness wheel.

Below is a list of additional sensory self-care activities to consider:

- Rub a worry stone or other small object between your fingers.
- Squeeze a stress ball.
- Listen to a podcast or nature sounds.
- Wrap your body in a blanket or lay under a weighted blanket.
- Use a yoga ball or a non-stable object to sit on while working.
- Use essential oils, incense, or aromatherapy.
- Play with kinetic sand, soft dough, or slime.
- Color in a coloring book or on blank paper.

- Walk barefoot in the grass or on sand.
- Guided meditations or visual meditations.
- Gentle body stretching or massage.
- Listen to the rain, wind, or sounds of nature.
- Slowly touch your thumb to each of your fingers in a repeating pattern.
- Gently tap your index finger in a repeating pattern on the chakra points of your body (forehead, throat, heart, sternum, stomach).

If the function of your current limiting behavior is sensory, these may be self-care activities that make sense for you and that you can easily incorporate into your every day. Remember that when sensory is a function, you want that physiological, sense-based approach to the self-care activity. In most cases, when you focus on your sense, you are also grounding yourself in the moment, which is also a calming and intentional relaxation strategy.

ESCAPE/AVOID ACTIVITIES

Escape activities are those that are already occurring, and avoidance are those that you evade. These are mostly associated with aversive stimuli or things that you don't like to do or people you don't want to see. When considering how to use escape and avoidance for self-care, you want to think about how you can escape and avoid in a healthy way. Everyone needs a break or a little time away from a difficult task or person.

Meditation Moments

One of the healthiest ways to break from a stressful world or to quickly gather your strength or a sense of calm before a challenging situation is to meditate. Meditation does not have to be an extensive, time-consuming action. Meditation can be as quick as one or two minutes. A short time for mindfulness helps pull yourself away from a difficult or taxing chore; it then allows you to reengage with the task with a better sense of wellbeing.

When first learning to meditate, many believe that it requires a full emptying of the mind, thoughtlessness. In fact, it's quite the opposite. Meditation is an active process that helps the mind to focus. There are different types of meditation, but two quick examples will be shared to begin a self-care practice.

The first meditation technique is quite easy. It's a strategy to help simplify your thoughts and reframe negative views. It can be used when you want to gain confidence or remove damaging self-talk. Sometimes the things we need to work to avoid or escape are our own limiting thoughts.

1. Find a quiet place to lay or sit with minimal or no distractions.
2. Sit or lie comfortably with your eyes closed.
3. Take several deep breaths, in through your nose and out through your mouth.
4. When you notice a thought appear, imagine that thought on top of a leaf.
5. The leaf with the thought on it is in the middle of a gently flowing river.
6. Allow the leaf and the thought to float carefully away down the river and out of your mind.
7. Each time a new thought enters, put it on a leaf and float it down the river.
8. It is okay for thoughts to come and go—be mindful of the thoughts and be careful to not allow them to linger.
9. Slowly reenter your actual space and open your eyes.

This meditation is intended to honor that thoughts are important and necessary but that they don't have to stay with you and you are in control of them. The second meditation technique is helpful when you want to "getaway." This meditation can be used to go to another place or time. It can provide a virtual escape.

1. Find a quiet place to lay or sit with minimal or no distractions.
2. Sit or lie comfortably with your eyes closed.
3. Take several deep breaths, in through your nose and out through your mouth.
4. Picture a beautiful scene of nature—a beach, the mountains, a flower-covered meadow, or a babbling brook.
5. Imagine all the details, the smells, the sounds, the feeling of the ground under your feet.
6. Take time to immerse yourself in the scene, walk along a mossy trail, feel the sand sink beneath your feet, feel cool snowflakes melt on your cheeks.
7. Slowly reenter your actual space and open your eyes.

After each of these meditations, you'll want to address the event that you escaped or avoided. Now that you are calm, relaxed, and have a clear mind, you can more carefully enter the challenging event. When you need to take a break or if you need to balance your wellness wheel with more nature, you can consider one of these two meditations.

Another strategy that may help if a function of limiting behaviors is escape or avoidance is simply unplugging. For many people, the constant pull of social media, instant access to information and news, and the immediacy of stimuli can be overwhelming. One of the best tools to escape or avoid these circumstances is to remove yourself from them by unplugging.

You can choose to schedule a specific time on a regular basis, or you can choose to randomly unplug or fully turn off your electronic devices, our phones, televisions, your tablets, all of them. You want to create silence and reduce the urge to check-in, post, or view.

It may not seem like much, but creating dedicated time throughout the week to unplug and either spend time in nature or in quiet can help to refocus you and your attention inward and toward more healthy self-care practices. Unplugging can also help you to escape or avoid the negative, complicated, or harmful influences that many feel when they are constantly plugged in.

Additional examples might include the following:

1. Break a task or activity down into smaller parts.
2. Choose between two similar activities.
3. Create a reminder or warning system before an activity.
4. Incorporate a timer to help create a time limit for the activity.
5. Digital detox by deleting phone apps from your phone.
6. Declutter an area of your home.

ATTENTION ACTIVITIES

Attention is one of the most common functions of behavior. As humans, we are social creatures. Most people crave opportunities to interrelate with others and engage in conversation, interaction, and community.

Sometimes people crave attention so much that they will engage in behaviors even if the outcome is unkind attention or hurtful attention. Have you ever know a child or an adult who even after getting in trouble and being reprimanded, even yelled at, will still do the same thing again? Often, that is attention-seeking behavior that can be very damaging to mental wellness.

Finding healthy and supportive ways to access attention is the key to a balanced self-care routine. Below are just a couple of examples that may help to provide healthy attention.

One strategy is called non-contingent reinforcement or non-contingent attention. It essentially means that attention is provided and it isn't contingent on a specific or target behavior occurring. Simply stated, it is not connected to the behavior. This is especially helpful if you notice that your behavior results in some challenging attention in return.

This can be accomplished by creating a schedule for chat times or check-in times with a select group of healthy people in your life. Throughout the day, you can schedule brief opportunities to receive healthy attention. You may want to let a few friends know that you'll be reaching out via phone, text, or instant message and just want to know how they are doing and what they are up to. The goal is just a quick, safe, and healthy conversation. These chat times can offer an appropriate means to gain attention.

There is now wider access to counseling and therapeutic supports that can be available via phone or text. If insurance covers it or if it is a low-cost option for you, these may be healthy opportunities for attention as well. If you have benefits through your employer, you may want to check if you have access to employee assistance programs or mental health benefits that provide opportunities to connect with a professional mental health provider.

Another strategy, especially for pet and animal lovers, is to gain attention from your furry friends who aren't concerned with why you want attention; they are just happy for some belly rubs. Similarly, schedule several breaks in the day, if this is feasible, and spend several quiet minutes with your pet. Even if a conversation with your puppy, cat, or ferret is essentially one-sided, it is still an opportunity to gain some attention.

A side benefit if you are a cat owner is that purrs also have healing effects. The frequency[1] at which cats purr has been known to have properties that can help heal soft tissue and bone, lowers stress, and can reduce the risk of heart disease. A cat's purr is a consistent pattern and frequency between 25 and 150 Hertz.

There are also activities now that allow children to read books to dogs. The concept is similar to scheduling some chat time with your pet. When a novice reader reads in front of a human audience, it can be intimidating and increase stressors and nerves. When a new reader reads in front of a dog, they are only receiving positive attention; there is no judgment or criticism from Fido. Just like scheduling your time with a pet for some attention, pets provide us healthy, accepting, and responsive attention when we need it.

So not only can some kitty conversations help to provide some necessary attention, they can even help heal us. And, though it may look silly to have a conversation with a dog, their attentive and responsive reaction may help provide the necessary attention to move past some unhealthy habits.

Some more examples of attention self-care actions are as follows:

1. Asking for validation or compliments.
2. Volunteering or doing community service.
3. Baking or making treats for friends/family/coworkers.
4. Hosting an event.
5. Becoming a mentor.
6. Giving a compliment to gain a compliment.
7. Saying a kind hello to a stranger and giving a smile.
8. Telling yourself three positive affirmations.
9. Hugging someone (who is prepared for a hug).

TANGIBLE ACTIVITIES

Tangible items are those things that you can hold on to or activities that you can enjoy. Tangible is all about having the things that make you happy. When tangible is a function, it is important to find time to enjoy what you have and what you can hold.

Two fairly easy things to consider for tangible are journaling and time-outs—not the time-outs that you're thinking of, but more like a date night or a girl's night. Not only will you get some positive attention, but you'll also fill your cup with a preferred activity. Quality time with quality people can help balance your wellness wheel.

The other great strategy is to keep a journal. There are several different kinds of journaling that you can consider, and any of them can help fulfill the need for tangible support. Journaling can not only support tangible benefits but also work as a stress reliever.

Consider trying one of the following if you are falling under the function of tangible:

1. Gratitude Journal

    This type of journaling is typically done two times a day, once in the morning and once in the evening. Each time you write at least three things that you are grateful for. It's okay to repeat items across the day or throughout the week as long as you are consistently keeping track of what makes you happy and grateful. Gratitude journals help you focus on the things that you are thankful for and potentially realize all the good that you possess in your life.

2. Morning Journal

    Morning journals are a time to focus each day with what you want to accomplish, what you dreamt at night, or what you are feeling first thing in the morning. This practice is intended to help you focus your mind on a single day and spend just a few moments each morning connecting yourself to your present circumstances. Again, the best practice is to focus on the positive.

3. To-Do Journal

    A to-do journal is just as it sounds. It is an opportunity to focus your intent on what you have to accomplish during that day or that week. It is an opportunity to create a list of intentions and goals to complete in a short period of time. It can be as simple as your chores and daily tasks or as complex as work goals that you want to finish or a DIY project. This journal is all about setting and accomplishing goals.

4. Done-with-It Journal

    The done-with-it journal is similar to the to-do journal, but it is more about tracking your accomplishments. This is typically done at the end of each day as a way to document what you finished. It is an opportunity to celebrate your completed goals and the tasks that you got done. If you like crossing off items on a to-do list, the done-with-it journal is a great option.

5. Vision Journal

    The vision journal is more long-term focused but can still be written each day. You begin the first journal entry with all of your visions, your wish lists, a vision of your dreams and future. Each day you can share how you accomplished getting closer to the goals or document that you reached a goal. You can continue to add to your wish list and even add images and drawings that showcase what you want.

Both journaling and time-out can help to fulfill your tangible needs. These activities can also help to reduce stress and provide opportunities to be mindful as well. The best thing about many of the activities listed across the function examples is that they may help to fill gaps or needs across many of the dimensions of wellness.

Here are a few more journaling prompts to try:

1. I am grateful for these strengths that I have. . .
2. A memory that I am thankful to remember is. . .
3. These are beautiful things that I see every day. . .
4. I feel comforted when I do. . .
5. This change _____ that I've made makes me happy because. . .

And, some additional examples of tangible self-care actions:

1. Search for sea shells, rocks, or unique leaves.
2. Create something new with recycled items.
3. Cook or bake something healthy.
4. Support a local business by buying from them.
5. Download a new app for your phone.
6. Put a puzzle together or take turns playing a game.
7. Make a vision board.
8. Go for a long walk.
9. Buy or pick yourself a bouquet of flowers.

At this time, you've had a few examples of how the functions of behavior can align with the eight dimensions of wellness. Now you can take these examples and begin to build out a more strategic plan that meets your needs. Take some time now to match self-care strategies to what you need to create a balanced wellness program.

Go to the blank self-care plan and fill in one column with self-care examples aligned to your function of behavior. There are some samples below to help you out.

You may find that there are dimensions that are more difficult to complete or that you have multiple self-care ideas that you can enter. For now, continue to add items to your list so that you have a toolbox of self-care strategies aligned to the function of the limiting behavior. When you feel that you have a dimension that is lacking or that you are struggling with, go back to your

Table 7.1 Matrix

	Sensory	Escape	Attention	Tangible
Section Three: Design				
Emotional			Ask a friend for a hug	
Spiritual				Donate to a charitable organization
Environmental				Plant a tree
Physical			Work out with a friend	
Intellectual	Listen to a podcast			
Social		Spend a night at home		
Occupational			Present a new idea at an upcoming meeting	
Financial				Save a penny in a paycheck

list and consider a new strategy or try a different strategy. At this point in your self-care journey, you just want to be sure that you have approaches to your self-care that align to the function and also meet the needs of the dimensions of wellness. This way, you have a number of ways that you can care for yourself in ways that you can feel confident will meet your needs.

SELF-CARE SYNERGY

This chapter started with the Greek term *Eunoia*, which means a *pure and well-balanced mind, a good spirit. Beautiful thinking.*

1. Imagine your personalized self-care plan as a house. Which self-care activities would you use to decorate each room and why?

2. Choose one activity from each function area and practice it with a family member or friend.
3. Design a lesson plan using at least one of the activities from this chapter.
4. Say no to one activity or event this week to allow yourself extra time to practice a self-care activity.

NOTE

1. https://www.scientificamerican.com/article/why-do-cats-purr/.

Chapter 8

Meraki—Greek

To do something with soul, creativity, or love; to put something of yourself into your work.

DO

This is the most difficult part of any plan—putting it into action. You have Discovered, Defined, and Designed; now, it is time to Do. One of the places that so many people get stuck in the action planning process is actually implementing the plan. This can be especially true for self-care activities since they require both action and self-reflection.

Remember when you learned about reinforcement earlier in the book? This is a great place in the process to think about not only the intrinsic motivation that you will likely gain from engaging in aligned self-care practices but also those external rewards that may help you stay motivated. After all, everyone needs a little extra nudge sometimes. You can create a plan to gain a preferred reward after you complete steps of an activity or complete the full activity. Just make sure that you keep your rewards healthy, too.

An example might be, if you are starting a new exercise routine, after you complete half of the activity, you can give yourself an extra-long break, especially if escape is a function for you, but you have to complete the other half of the routine. If you are trying to get outside to walk more, add a fun game to the activity to encourage motivation like a scavenger hunt or an "I spy" activity. If you are working on spending less time on social media, create small goals like during the first week you are on social media for two hours a day, the next week only one, the next week only thirty minutes until you are no longer reliant on social media. As a reward, perhaps at the end of the week, you treat yourself to a streaming movie.

Starting new routines and developing new habits may require two things: a step-up process and a reward process. In behavior analysis, this is often referred to as shaping. Shaping means that you are reinforcing successive approximations toward the end goal. For the exercise example, consider that your long-term goal is to do at least three hours of low-impact exercise a week. Currently, you are able to do about forty-five minutes to an hour. For two weeks, you can have the goal of one hour and earn a reward after that hour. Then, two weeks after that, the new goal is two hours followed up with a reward until you've worked up to the three-hour goal.

To focus on your goal and build in a reinforcer to help maintain your success, consider using a process of If-Then-When-Earn. It's a process to help build your self-care routine so that you can plan your goals and your motivation systems. It goes like this: *If* I do this, *then* this will happen and *when* this happens, I'll *earn* this.

Let's put it into action.

You can add, refine, and update your goal as often as needed. You want to be steadfast with your goals but flexible about how you get there. Remember that you may adjust your self-care activities as you progress and grow, as long as they align to the function of your behavior. But you want to maintain

Table 8.1

	Section Four: Do
If-Then-When-Earn	
If: enter your self-care activity aligned to a function of behavior	If I do this_____
Then: describe your initial goal	Then this will happen_____
When: Write your goal again	When this happens_____
Earn: enter in what award you'll earn when you meet your goal	I'll earn this_____

an ultimate goal. You may create smaller goals along the way as you shape toward the overall goal.

But, getting to the goal is not the end. Now you want to maintain that goal across time. The best way to know if you can maintain the goal for the long haul is by beginning to reduce the reinforcement that occurs after. So, now you are slowly going to reduce the "break" that you earn as part of the exercise program. If you can continue to maintain that three-hour-a-week goal, you have begun the process of what behavior analysts would call reinforcement fading.

Reinforcement fading is a process to reduce the reliance on external rewards. It is really when the action or behavior itself becomes the reward. The behavior is providing the functional outcome. This is especially important when you think about self-care. If you have determined the accurate function for your limiting behavior(s) and you have aligned self-care strategies that fulfill the dimensions of wellness, that intrinsic motivation should take over and exercise should become the reward in and of itself. For many of your habits that is likely already the case—now that you are working on developing new and healthier habits, you are working toward that automaticity of enjoyment.

You are working to find what the psychologist Mihaly Csikszentmihalyi called Flow[1]. Flow is a state of optimal experience and optimal development. It is best described as those times that you are so engrossed in an activity that you are lost in it. You almost lose time because you are doing something you are both good at and enjoy. Your self-care should help you to reach a state of flow eventually.

Another important consideration is what behaviorists call generalizing. This requires that the behavior, in this case, your self-care routine, can be maintained across multiple settings and across people. Consider how you will maintain that exercise routine if you go on vacation. Can you schedule the time or incorporate into your daily activities? Would the rewards need to be reestablished temporarily during that short time? It's okay if that is the case; the important thing is to continue to support your overall wellness.

One strategy that may help you as you begin your self-care plan, as you work on maintenance, and as you fade reinforcement or generalize your routine is to monitor what you do. Data help to tell the story of your success. Remember, data collection does not need to be complicated or time-consuming. In some cases, you may be able to use those online tools or applications that can help with some of the healthy habit monitoring.

The best strategy to use is self-monitoring. You are the constant observer of your behavior. It would likely be too difficult to have a family member or a friend to follow you around all day, every day, to watch you and track your habits. But you are always with you. You can track your behaviors. By collecting ongoing data, you can see if growth has occurred, which could be an increase or a decrease in the behavior depending on the goal.

As mentioned, keep it simple. If you are working on eating healthier, you can keep a food journal or track your calories using notes or a mobile phone application. If you are exercising more, your phone may already help track heart rate and steps taken per day. You can also create a simple tracking sheet where you write down what exercise you did, when you started, and when you stopped. If you are going to reduce your spending habits, your bank may have a budgeting plan that you can access online or you can download a free budget template online.

SELF-CARE SYNERGY

This chapter started with the Greek term *Meraki*, meaning t*o do something with soul, creativity, or love; to put something of yourself into your work.*

1. Turn an everyday chore into something more mindful. If you are doing laundry, take time to feel the fabric of each piece of clothing as you fold them. If you are cooking dinner, taste each component of the meal as it is being prepared. If you are cleaning, sing a song to help pass the time.
2. Reflect on when you have experienced a state of flow. What were you doing? Why were you so engrossed in it? Who was present or not present during that time?
3. If you are able, download at least one app on your phone or mobile device that you can use to help track data.
4. Take a break. Right now. Just take a deep breath, roll your shoulders down and back. Relax the muscles in your face. Relax.

NOTE

1. Nakamura, J. and Csikszentmihalyi, M. (2014) The Concept of Flow. In *Flow and the Foundations of Positive Psychology*. Dordrecht: Springer. https://link.springer.com/book/10.1007/978-94-017-9088-8.

Chapter 9

Kalo—Hawaiian

There are no limits

Self-Care for Students

PAYING IT FORWARD

The best part of any successful plan is paying it forward. Now that you have the steps for success, consider how all of this can apply to your other role, educator. You likely work with some students who struggle to develop their own health habits or who have experienced challenges in life from which they could benefit from self-care.

You may have even helped students learn skills like taking a deep breath, walking away from a conflict, or how to make friends. All of these are what educators will call social-emotional learning (SEL) skills, and what you know are also self-care strategies. You have likely created lesson plans and classroom activities to help teach these skills to the students that you care for.

Below are a few examples of how you can share your self-care and wellness strategies with your students and in your classroom.

CANDLE BLOWOUT

Use engaging and even fun activities to teach how and when to take deep breaths. People love blowing out the candles on their birthday cake. One strategy to learn how to take deep and relaxing breaths is to "blow out the birthday candles". Have the student(s) close their eyes and pretend there is a big birthday cake in front of them, full of lit candles. They can even make a wish before taking a deep breath in and blowing all the air out, just like if they were trying to extinguish birthday candles.

Practicing this can help students to redirect their frustration or anxiousness toward a more positive activity. This can help provide a short period of mindfulness and visual meditation as students imagine the scene. And it creates a reason to take in and release a deep healthy breath.

CROSSING THE MERIDIAN

A student who may need to take a short brain break and refocus can do an activity called crossing the meridian. This is another helpful grounding and mindful moment that also has some brain science behind it[1,2,3]. Crossing the midline of the body or the invisible middle equator of that splits the left from the right side and is said to help the two hemispheres of the brain work together.

By having students do short, simple activities like hold their arms up in front of them and then cross their left hand over their right and then in reverse may help to create a sense of calm and also focus. This body crossing activity can be done with the legs as well. While we typically cross the meridian of our bodies on a regular basis throughout the day, taking a moment to focus on the activity can create a short break and an opportunity to refocus the mind on a mindful moment to stimulate each side of the body and brain.

PROPRIOCEPTIVE POSITIONS

Proprioception is a fancy way to say, feeling our bodily movements. For students, it is incredibly important to understand how the positions of our bodies impact the world around us. Helping students to both understand proprioception and practice activities to activate their sensory systems can be incredibly beneficial.

This can be especially helpful for active students, students with a lot of energy and students who are impacted by anxiety. You can play a quick game of Simon Says with nose touches, toe touches, and tummy patting. You can have students gently push their hands against a wall. Have the student give themselves a tight hug and then release. These activities can also be combined with visual meditations providing both sensory stimulation and mindfulness.

TUCK LIKE AN ARMADILLO

Similar to proprioceptive positions, tucking like an armadillo provides sensory stimulation and mindfulness. This also provides the ability to practice positive self-talk and create a sense of calm and influence, and pretending can also activate brain stimulation that helps to redirect anxious feelings.

You want to start by explaining that when armadillos get nervous, anxious, or scared, they tuck their bodies away in their shells to protect themselves. You can show a student what that looks like by making your body small and tucking in your arms and legs, then have them practice tucking into a small little ball.

Then share that armadillos can't stay like that for long, so they get brave and big. Unwrap yourself and make your body big with arms and legs outstretched. Have the student practice this as well. Students can then practice tucking and getting big while also taking deep breaths—a deep breath in to tuck and a deep breath out when untucking.

This activity combines deep breathing, proprioception, visualization, reframing thoughts, and creating a sense of calm and control. Even if there is not a lot of physical space, students can practice by tightening their body while taking a deep breath and releasing their body while letting out the deep breath.

COUNTDOWN TO CALM

A simple grounding activity often used when someone is experiencing a panic attack or severe anxiety is to use a 5, 4, 3, 2, 1 strategy. This is an activity to help with emotional regulation. To do this, the student would take a deep breath and find five things they can see, four things they can hear, three things they can smell, two things they can feel, and one thing they can taste. This practice provides an opportunity to practice mindfulness and ground their senses in reality rather than the what-ifs that are creating the feelings of restlessness.

All of these activities can be used with students and people of all ages. You can make minor adjustments based on age and developmental level. You can practice the same self-care activities when you are feeling out of balance. Remember that you are the model of wellness for your students.

The most important thing for students and for you is to begin to recognize the connection between the body and the mind. The two systems function in collaboration. When one is out of balance the other likely will struggle. If you are in pain, your mind may produce more stress chemicals. When your brain is focused on negative thoughts, your body may tense up and tighten.

To help students and adults learn about the connection, it is vital to begin recognizing where feelings start in the body and label that location and feeling. For example, when people feel frustrated, they can clench their fists or feel a flutter in their stomach. When people feel scared, they can freeze or tense their muscles. When people are sad or angry, they can feel a lump in their throat. Each of these feelings is connected to a place in the body that is also impacted and that physiological response may be the first sign of the psychological feeling.

If you can recognize or help students to recognize the connection, that is, "if this happens in my body, I am feeling this," then everyone will be more equipped to engage in a self-care activity early enough to reduce the overall impact of the stressor. If you couple that with the knowledge of what the function of the behavior is, like when a frustrated person uses inappropriate language which is most often rewarded with attention from others, then you have the recipe for creating a solid self-care plan.

SELF-CARE SYNERGY

This chapter started with a Hawaiian term *Kalo*, meaning *there are no limits*.

1. If you had no limits in life, what would be different? What would be the same? Write a story or journal about your life with no limits.
2. Practice each of the student examples from this chapter. Are they helpful for you? How could you integrate them into your overall self-care strategies?

3. Teach one of the strategies from this chapter to a family member, friend, or student. Go through each of the steps and have a discussion after to talk about whether or not it helped and why.
4. Draw a diagram of the body. Circle the location on the body that you first notice feeling happy, feeling upset, feeling scared, feeling love, and so on. Create or print a blank cartoon body and create a lesson plan to do this activity with your students to help them recognize how emotions are connected to physical feelings.

NOTES

1. Bradshaw, J. L., Spataro, J. A., Harris, M., Nettleton, N. C., and Bradshaw, J. (1988) Crossing the midline by four- to eight-year-old children. *Neuropsychologia* 26, 221–235. doi: 10.1016/0028-3932(88)90076-0.

2. Cermak, S. A., and Ayres, A. J. (1984) Crossing the body midline in learning-disabled and normal children. *American Journal of Occupational Therapy* 38, 35–39. doi: 10.5014/ajot.38.1.35.

3. Michell, D., and Wood, N. (1999) An investigation of midline crossing in three-year-old children. *Physiotherapy* 85, 607–615. doi: 10.1016/S0031-9406(05)66041-5.

Conclusion

SELF-CARE IS A PRACTICE

You have accomplished the most essential part of your self-care journey: you have dedicated time and energy to becoming a better you and therefore a better educator. Through this first step, you have altered the balance of your wellness for the better.

Throughout each chapter of this book, you have created a self-care story. You have built layer upon layer of learning about yourself and your needs. Like the first few weeks of a new school year, you have focused on the most vital parts of learning—getting to know the individual needs of each student. This time, you were the student.

You reflected on your habits and routines. You observed your days and behaviors. You collected data and paid attention to patterns. You determined balanced strategies to create a plan that works for you.

It has been said that yoga is called a practice because it is ongoing; it is never perfected. Your self-care journey is also a practice. You have the opportunity now to focus more on what works and does not work for you and make small changes that are best aligned to the why, the function of those behaviors.

Throughout each chapter, you gained a better sense of building a strategic plan. Sure, you could continue to just try every new fad or all the different wellness trends that are out there, but much like in the classroom, if you don't tailor the support to the student, you run the risk of wasting time, money, and resources.

At the end of each chapter were opportunities for you to reflect. The self-care synergy activities were all aligned to the eight dimensions of wellness and the four functions of behavior. If you ever need to adjust your strategy or update your plan, consider that you have all the tools you need to be a *selfist*. You are armed with the power to practice a well-balanced life.

There are just a few more important lessons to consider on your self-care journey, lessons that may help you as you find the need to find balance again or if you ever feel off balance. These are lessons learned from the classroom and on the yoga mat. Much like your classroom rules, consider these your self-care rules.

BE OBSERVANT

Pay attention. It is easy for old and unhealthy habits and routines to drift back to us or around us. Pay attention. When you observe that balance is being tipped, go back to your self-care plan and determine if the same process can be revisited or if a new plan should be devised.

In yoga, it is taught that you should pay attention to how your body feels and listen to your body. It is not about pushing yourself, but about listening and adjusting, and being observant.

In the classroom, it is the same. You observe. You scan the room. You listen and you attend to what is happening in each moment. In the classroom, it is often called with-it-ness, the ability to know what is happening and respond accordingly.

Understand that behavior takes time and consistency to change. You will need to continue your self-care practices until that drift to old patterns is no longer there. There is no set time or number of events that occurs, so you have to continue to observe.

There is an adage in the behavioral field that for every year that you have engaged in a behavior, it could take that many months of *consistent* intervention and reinforcement to change. So, if you engaged in your limiting behavior for five years, it could take up to five months to make a significant change. And that is with consistency!

Continue to pay attention to your practice and allow yourself the greatest amount of consistency possible. It won't be perfect; nothing is. You can create the circumstances for healthy habits to take shape if you continue to observe and adjust.

BE FLEXIBLE

When offered a chance to attend a yoga class, the most common response is, "I'm not flexible." Yoga is not about becoming a human pretzel. In fact, it is truly the opposite. It is about feeling the pose that you are in and adjusting if necessary.

Flexibility is the ability to bend without breaking. Consider those balls that you are balancing as part of your everyday juggle. Even with some of those areas of your life being fragile and delicate, you work to manage them without breaking any.

In the classroom, the ability to pivot, adjust, and be nimble is ongoing. There are seldom moments when agility isn't required. There are a few times that plans don't require tweaking.

Your self-care journey will require the flexibility to bend. You may find times when parts of the plan no longer work or new challenges are thrown at you. You have the tools to determine how to bend, how to tweak, and how to sustain that balance.

BE DILIGENT

In the classroom you can't let your guard down. You have to be attentive. You have to be assiduous in order to meet the needs of all learners and requirements.

On the yoga mat, it is said that the hardest pose to hold is likely the one you need the most. This means that the greatest challenges are likely to become our greatest successes. Those things that we'd like to avoid the most may actually provide the highest growth.

Be diligent with your self-care. Make the time. Use your plan. Hold yourself to your goals.

BE PATIENT

If you have ever experienced a student that is difficult, you likely learned that patience can go a long way to helping you and the student be successful. It is easy to let our emotions take over. It is easy to get lost in a moment of unkindness or irritation.

Be patient with yourself. You are learning or relearning to take care of yourself as part of this self-care journey. You will slip back into old ways. You will find negative emotions growing louder. You will tell yourself you can't, you shouldn't, and you aren't worth it.

But you are and you can. Yoga teaches us to accept what we can do in each moment, to not compare to another person or even one side of the body to the other. Each pose is it's own. Each position is a chance to learn and soften.

Each part of this self-care process is an opportunity for you to learn, to grow, to nurture. Each dimension is a chance to experience something new. Each day is the chance to practice care for yourself.

BE KIND

The golden rule in the classroom, on the yoga mat, and in life is to treat others the way you want to be treated. This requires that you treat yourself with the kindness that you want to see in others. It starts with you.

In the behavior world, it is said that you can't control anyone else; the only thing that you can control is how you respond. Respond to yourself with kindness. You are in control of how you treat yourself. Treat yourself with kindness. Be gentle when you fall, be strong when you are scared, be kind when are healing.

Whether it is challenging behaviors in the classroom or difficult times in your life—you have the skills, the process, and the plan to manifest your happy.

Appendix

Self-Care Plan

This is your self-care plan. You can fill it in as you read through the book or you can complete it once you have finished the book. This is your plan.

The plan is intended to help you organize your thoughts, understand your behaviors and habits and align your needs to create a plan that is personalized and specific to you.

This plan may only need to be done one time for you to reap the benefits of strategic self-care or you may need to revise the plan several times or revisit it throughout your life.

The most important piece is that you honor yourself by being true to you and true to your hopes and wishes for a fulfilling life.

Begin Here

Map of Impact

2. What happens right before the beahvior?

3. What happens right after the behavior?

1. Enter a limiting behavior

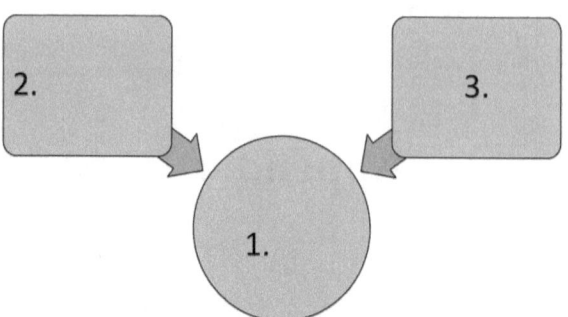

Section One: Discover
1. Why are you investing in yourself?
2. How will investing in yourself help you as an educator?

List three *harmful* habits that you currently have.	1. 2. 3.
List three *healthy/helpful* habits that you currently have.	1. 2. 3.
What are some ways to increase your healthy/helpful habits? List any strategies you have tried or considered in the past or new ideas that you'd like to try.	

	Write down the typical pattern of your day
Morning	
Afternoon	
Evening	
During your day, what are the people, places, items, or activities that *don't* bring you much happiness?	
List three people that bring you joy.	1. 2. 3.
List three places that bring you joy.	1. 2. 3.
List three items that bring you joy.	1. 2. 3.
List three activities that bring you joy.	1. 2. 3.

Section Two: Define

Write the operational definition for the limiting behavior you are going to monitor.

Section Two Cont'd: Define

Create an ABC chart for one week. Choose a *single* behavior, list and write it in the 'B' column. All week track what happens right before ('A' column) and right after ('B' column) that behavior.			What trends or patterns do you notice in the 'C' (consequence) column?
A	**B**	**C**	
	e.g. too much screentime		

Section Two Cont'd: Define

Frequency (e.g. III II III)		M	T	W	Th	F	S	Su
	6-9am							
	9-12pm							
	12-3pm							
	3-6pm							
	6-9pm							
	9-12pm							
	12-3am							
	3-1am							

Duration (e.g. 3pm -4:32pm)	Start time: _____	Stop time: _____
	Start time: _____	Stop time: _____
	Start time: _____	Stop time: _____
	Start time: _____	Stop time: _____
	Start time: _____	Stop time: _____
	Start time: _____	Stop time: _____
	Start time: _____	Stop time: _____
	Start time: _____	Stop time: _____

Latency (e.g. 1:24 – 1:33)	Time Instruction Given	Time Behavior Begins

Section Two Cont'd: Define

Respond to the questions below.

Overview
1. What is my current limiting behavior?
2. When does it occur most often?
3. How long does it typically last?
4. What is the outcome of the limiting behavior?

Antecedents
1. What was the most commonly occurring consequence when collecting ABC data?
2. What does that commonly occurring consequence help me understand about the limiting behavior?

Consequences
1. Is the consequence most often a person or interaction with a person?
2. Is the consequence most often getting away from someone or something?
3. Is the consequence typically gaining an item or object?

Data Collection
1. The data collection helped me realize the behavior occurs frequently?
2. The data collection helped me realize the behavior occurs for periods of time?
3. The data collection helped me realize the behavior occurs in this pattern?

Appendix

	Section Two Cont'd: Define
Hypothesis statement for the limiting behavior	When (describe the common setting/location or environmental factors that the behavior occurs in) _____ I will (write in the limiting behavior) _____ in order to gain (add the *ONE most likely* function based on your data collection and the questions you answered above) Attention ☐ Escape/Avoid ☐ Tangible ☐ Sensory ☐

Section Three: Design

In this example, there are samples in each of the columns of the Self-Care Design. You will only need to complete on full column. For example, if the function of your limiting behavior is Escape/Avoidance, you'll add a self-care example down the Escape column for each of the dimensions of wellness.

	Sensory	Escape	Attention	Tangible
Emotional				
Spiritual				
Environmental				
Physical				
Intellectual				
Social				
Occupational				
Financial				

Section Four: Do	
If-Then-When-Earn **If**: enter your self-care activity aligned to a function of behavior **Then**: describe your initial goal **When**: Write your goal again **Earn**: enter in what award you'll earn when you meet your goal	If I do this_____ Then this will happen_____ When this happens_____ I'll earn this_____

Personal Reflection	
Use this area of the plan to reflect, connect, and grow. You can take notes, you can write your mantra or things you are grateful for. You can plan or create new goals. You can add plans on how to integrate self-care in to your education practices. This is your section.	

Endnote References
(In order of appearance)

1. Ingersoll, R. M., Merrill, E., Stuckey, D., and Collins, G. (2018) Seven Trends: The Transformation of the Teaching Force – Updated October 2018. *CPRE Research Reports.* Retrieved from https://repository.upenn.edu/cpre_researchreports/108.
2. https://pdkpoll.org/results.
3. https://pdkpoll.org/results.
4. https://www.samhsa.gov/.
5. An internet resource developed by Green, C. D. http://www.yorku.ca/dept/psych/classics/author.htm. Toronto, Ontario: York University. ISSN 1492-3713.
6. https://www.medicalnewstoday.com/articles/66840#1.
7. https://www.authentichappiness.sas.upenn.edu/home.
8. Coles, N. A., Larsen, J. T., and Lench, H. C. (2019) A meta-analysis of the facial feedback literature: Effects of facial feedback on emotional experience are small and variable. *Psychological Bulletin*, 145(6), 610–651. http://dx.doi.org/10.1037/bul0000194.
9. https://www.cdc.gov/violenceprevention/childabuseandneglect/acestudy/index.html.
10. https://www.cdc.gov/violenceprevention/childabuseandneglect/acestudy/about.html.
11. https://www.cdc.gov/violenceprevention/childabuseandneglect/aces/fastfact.html.
12. https://dickmalott.com/.
13. https://www.apa.org/monitor/2010/01/little-albert.
14. Skinner, B. F. (1959) *Cumulative Record.* New York: Appleton Century Crofts.
15. Skinner, B. F. (1974) *About Behaviorism*, New York: Knopf.

16. https://thoughtcatalog.com/brianna-wiest/2017/11/this-is-what-self-care-really-means-because-its-not-all-salt-baths-and-chocolate-cake/Albert Szent-Gyorgyi.
17. https://www.scientificamerican.com/article/why-do-cats-purr/.
18. Nakamura, J., and Csikszentmihalyi, M. (2014) The Concept of Flow. In *Flow and the Foundations of Positive Psychology*. Dordrecht: Springer. https://link.springer.com/book/10.1007/978-94-017-9088-8.
19. Bradshaw, J. L., Spataro, J. A., Harris, M., Nettleton, N. C., and Bradshaw, J. (1988) Crossing the midline by four to eight year old children. *Neuropsychologia* 26, 221–235. doi: 10.1016/0028-3932(88)90076-0.
20. Cermak, S. A., and Ayres, A. J. (1984) Crossing the body midline in learning-disabled and normal children. *American Journal of Occupational Therapy* 38, 35–39. doi: 10.5014/ajot.38.1.35.
21. Michell, D., and Wood, N. (1999) An investigation of midline crossing in three-year-old children. *Physiotherapy* 85, 607–615. doi: 10.1016/S0031-9406(05)66041-5.

About the Author

Jenna Sage is an enlightened emotional influencer who welds the fabric of life through storytelling, builds knowledge through collaborative resource mining, and guides teaming through teachable moments.

She has worked in multiple capacities in the field of education for nearly twenty-five years. Sage earned a PhD in Special Education, specializing in systems change processes. She is a practicing behavior analyst and a professional business and life coach. She is also a consultant, a speaker, and a writer focusing on helping professionals apply the science of behavior pragmatically, meaningfully, and with sustainability.

www.ingramcontent.com/pod-product-compliance
Lightning Source LLC
Chambersburg PA
CBHW032030230426
43671CB00005B/260